AN INTRODUCTION TO
Social Medicine

AN INTRODUCTION TO

Social Medicine

Thomas McKeown

M.D. Ph.D. D.Phil. F.R.C.P.
Professor of Social Medicine
University of Birmingham

C. R. Lowe

M.D. Ph.D. F.R.C.G.P. F.F.C.M.
Professor of Social and Occupational Medicine
Welsh National School of Medicine, Cardiff

Second edition
Second printing

BLACKWELL SCIENTIFIC PUBLICATIONS
OXFORD LONDON EDINBURGH MELBOURNE

© 1966, 1974 Blackwell Scientific Publications
Osney Mead, Oxford,
8 John Street, London WCI,
9 Forrest Road, Edinburgh,
P.O. Box 9, North Balwyn, Victoria, Australia.

ISBN 0 632 09310 2

First published 1966
Second printing 1968
Second edition 1974
Second printing 1977

Printed in Great Britain by
Offset Lithography by
Billing & Sons Limited,
Guildford, London and Worcester.

CONTENTS

Control of Environment

PART III—SERVICES

Evolution of Health and Related Social Services

Present-Day Health and Related Social Services

INTRODUCTION

In most branches of biology and medicine the nature of the subject matter is reflected accurately in the title. Anatomy is concerned with structure, physiology with function and obstetrics with childbearing; and whatever differences of opinion there may be about methods of instruction, teachers can usually take it for granted that they are talking about the same thing. This is an assumption which the writer on social medicine cannot make, and it is essential at the outset to clarify the use of the term.

In contemporary usage social medicine has two meanings, one broad and ill-defined, the other more restricted and precise. In the broad sense, social medicine is an expression of the humanitarian tradition in medicine, and people frequently read into it any interpretation consistent with their own aspirations and interests. Thus it may be identified with humane care of patients, prevention of disease, administration of medical services; indeed with almost any subject in the extensive field of health and welfare. But in the more restricted sense in which we shall be using the term, social medicine is concerned with a body of knowledge and methods of obtaining knowledge appropriate to a discipline.

This discipline may be said to comprise (a) *epidemiology* and (b) *the study of the medical needs of society, or, in the contemporary shorthand, medical care.*

These subjects were a relatively late development in medicine. Until the nineteenth century medical service comprised little more than the care of patients who sought the assistance of the doctor. It was the threat of infection which finally led to recognition of the need for another approach. Diseases such as smallpox, cholera and typhoid could not be treated effectively in individual patients; but they could be prevented by measures directed to the community as a whole.

The new developments in the second half of the nineteenth century had two important features. One was investigation of disease by epidemiological methods; the other was an interest in the medical needs of society, for example in protection against smallpox, in control of the physical environment and in provision of fever hospitals. These features were adopted, not because our predecessors were exceptionally perceptive, but because they offered the only feasible approach to the predominant problem of infection. It was not a coincidence that public medical services were introduced at the time when epidemiological methods were first applied widely to the study of disease.

In technologically advanced countries the problem of infection is today much smaller, but the two features of social medicine are as necessary as ever. Indeed their full significance is only beginning to be realized. In almost all branches of medicine investigation based on groups rather than on individuals is an indispensable complement to the traditional methods of laboratory and clinical research. And acceptance of national responsibility for medical services, far from resolving the problems of medical care, has revealed the paucity of data required for their solution.

This book is concerned only with the second of these subjects, that is with the medical needs of society or, more briefly, medical care. Since departments of social medicine teach both epidemiology and medical care this may seem a surprising restriction but the reasons for it appear to us compelling. The two subjects, although related, are essentially different, and it is undesirable to attempt to cover them in the same book, particularly if the discussion of epidemiology includes not only its scope and techniques but also its contributions to knowledge, for example of specific diseases. It is on these grounds that the present book has been limited to the medical care theme, on the assumption that students will have access to other instruction on epidemiology. Nevertheless it may be useful to provide in this introduction a brief account of the scope of both subjects.

Epidemiology

The following developments can be recognized in the evolution of epidemiology, identified by the use of population methods in the study of different problems.

1. Infectious disease. Epidemiological methods were first employed extensively to investigate the distribution and causes of the infections and until well into the present century this was almost their sole use.

2. Non-infectious disease. Although population methods were used earlier in nutritional and toxicological studies, it is only during the past few decades that they have been applied widely in investigation of non-infectious disease. It was above all the early (in this context) and impressive findings concerning the multiple effects of smoking which stimulated this development, but it has been extended rapidly to a wide range of problems such as chronic bronchitis, hypertension, coronary artery disease and abnormalities associated with reproduction.

3. Human biology. Investigation of growth and development in populations preceded the modern recognition of the scope of epidemiology. The study of intelligence, mainly in school children, also anticipated by many years the contemporary interest in epidemiology, but there is perhaps no subject which illustrates better the need for improved data and the more rigorous analysis that can now be provided. Reproduction and arterial pressure are other examples of fields in which the same methods have been applied successfully in investigation of normal variation.

4. Medical and surgical procedures. Yet another important development was the recognition that clinical experience does not provide a sufficient basis for evaluation of medical and surgical procedures and that both preventive and therapeutic measures require assessment, ideally in populations assigned at random to study and control groups. Among the best known examples of this approach are the clinical trial of vaccines used in prevention of diseases such as poliomyelitis and measles. In the same context reference should also be made to the need for epidemiological appraisal of the harm which results from medical procedures. With the increasing complexity and power of methods of investigation and treatment it seems inevitable that these risks will increase and it is a challenge to the epidemiologist to help in assessment and, so far as possible, elimination of the dangers.

5. Validity of observations. In recent years epidemiologists have begun to demonstrate and measure the range of errors associated with common laboratory and clinical procedures. Many of these are the result of observer error, or, more charitably, observer variation, for example in interpretation of X-rays and ECG's. Very recently the use of automated methods and of the computer has provided a more

accurate picture of variation in chemical estimations of the constituents of blood or urine.

6. Health services. The applications outlined above illustrate a gradual, and recently fairly rapid, evolution of concepts concerning the uses of population methods in biology and medicine. The field which remains to be cultivated extensively is that of health services. The character of health services has been determined hitherto by multiple influences, including their history, public demand, political considerations and the doctor's impression of what is good for his patients; services have not been planned in the light of an accurate appraisal of needs and the optimum deployment of resources. However the volume of work is increasing and the subjects under investigation include screening in medical care, health information systems, organization of medical institutions such as hospitals, health centres and polyclinics as well as management and economic problems. Moreover the attack is not limited to the study of existing practices and institutions but includes assessment of the health problems confronting society, reasons for improvement in health, appraisal of medical measures, the planning and management of health services and the measurement of their effectiveness. Needless to say, epidemiology is only one of several disciplines required for the study of such complex problems.

The medical needs of society ('Medical care')

This subject may be said to be concerned broadly with appraisal of the medical problems of society and the means at our disposal for solving them. It is needed because the role of medicine in society is immensely complex, and cannot be understood without some knowledge of the problems of sickness and death, of the wide range of influences which contribute to health, and of the services through which our resources are mobilized. These themes are the subject matter of the three divisions of this book: Problems; Means; and Services.

Part I attempts to assess broadly the nature of the medical task. It considers first the extent and causes of past improvement in health, and so places medical achievement in perspective in relation to other influences (such as a rising standard of living) which have also contributed (Chapter 1). Chapter 2 then examines the effects of the advances on the problems confronting medicine and discusses some of the ethical issues associated with contemporary health problems. Chapter 3 considers the possibility that the decline of mortality has resulted in deterioration of the genetic constitution of the population. The last three chapters of Part I are concerned with contemporary health problems, both national and international.

Part II provides an appraisal of the means which can be used to improve health. In principle they are of two kinds: control of inheritance and control of environment. Chapter 7 considers the difficulties associated with the control of human reproduction and the reasons why it has so far been of little practical importance in relation to disease. Attention is then focused on other influences, and a broad distinction is made between personal and environmental measures. The former are taken to comprise all influences directed to the individual, and so defined include the practice of clinical medicine. Since an evaluation of clinical methods is considered in clinical teaching, the discussion of personal measures is restricted to three approaches which are already or potentially very significant: immunization; screening; and modification of personal behaviour.

The environmental measures discussed in Part II are those which can be implemented by public action, largely, and sometimes wholly, without the co-operation of individuals. Among the more important are the control of food, water, air, animal vectors of disease, home and place of work.

It should perhaps be emphasized that the discussion of environmental measures is not concerned with the techniques used to control the environment. It does not, for example, describe the means by which the atmosphere is cleaned or water purified. These methods are highly technical; most of them are not the concern of doctors, and those which are, are used mainly by specialists. The object of the discussion is rather to give a broad view of the tools which are available or are potentially available, for the improvement of health.

Part III considers the services through which medical knowledge and resources are applied. The first section discusses the evolution of health and related social services, and the way in which their development influenced their post war organization. The second section deals with the present day pattern of services. Chapters 24 and 25 describe the health and social services since their reorganization in 1974 and 1972 respectively; the remaining chapters are concerned with the services available to special groups such as children, the handicapped and the elderly. The aim here is to estimate the needs of different sections of the population, to describe the services and to consider whether they are adequate.

ACKNOWLEDGMENT

We are indebted to George Allen & Unwin Ltd for permission to reproduce some of the material in chapters 1–4 of *Medicine in Modern Society* by T. McKeown.

PART I
Problems

1 · ASSESSMENT OF IMPROVEMENT IN HEALTH

In the year 1818 Shelley left England for the last time, accompanied by his wife, his two children, Byron's mistress, Byron's child and two nursemaids. A year later his wife gave birth to a third child. By the time of Shelley's death four years later three of the four children were dead. Mortality of this order was not restricted to the children of poets with a predilection for foreign travel. It was an accurate reflection of the prevailing death rates, a situation vividly portrayed in nineteenth century novels.

The improvement in health which has occurred since then is well illustrated by the increase in expectation of life (table 1). In 1693 Halley prepared the first 'life tables' (for Breslau) which show per 1000 individuals born alive the numbers expected to live to different ages. At that time approximately half would survive to age 10. Similar data are available for England and Wales since 1838, when half could expect to live to 40. By 1970 rather more than half could expect to live to 70.

To assess the extent and causes of improvement in health more precisely it is necessary to clarify objectives and define indices of achievement. This is more difficult in medicine than in most other public activities. A broadcasting system should entertain and inform; a postal service should deliver mail quickly and reliably; but it is not possible to state medical objectives which are equally clear and acceptable. Few people would quarrel with the view that it is desirable to prevent illness and premature death; but some would feel that these aims are not ambitious enough, that it is also necessary to prolong the normal life span and promote positive health. Unfortunately these objectives are not yet within reach; and for the purpose of assessing past achievement the only ones that can be accepted without reservation are prevention of sickness, disability and premature death and alleviation of the suffering caused by illness. In relation to these aims the most suitable indices are sickness and death rates.

Table 1. Expectation of life at different periods

	Number surviving out of 1,000 live born males				
Age	1693*	1838–54†	1891–1900†	1920–22†	1970†
0	1,000	1,000	1,000	1,000	1,000
5	582	724	750	870	976
10	531	690	734	857	974
15	505	673	725	849	973
20	481	652	712	837	968
30	426	595	673	805	959
40	356	532	616	763	947
50	275	456	531	699	909
60	191	356	410	588	802
70	110	223	247	395	563
80		80	82	150	236

* Halley's life tables (Breslau).
† From English life tables.

About morbidity (sickness) it should be said at once that even today the data are limited, and for periods before the present century there is no reliable information. The reason is clear: many non-fatal illnesses never come to medical attention, and some which do present formidable problems of diagnosis and classification. Until recently knowledge of morbidity was almost restricted to a group of 'notifiable diseases', such as smallpox, tuberculosis and diphtheria, with two things in common: they usually present in recognizable form; and their occurrence is of considerable practical importance to public medical authorities.

Because knowledge of sickness is so deficient, assessment of the improvement in health must be based chiefly on information about death; this is available for England and Wales since 1838, when births, deaths and cause of death were first registered nationally. In Sweden birth and death rates were recorded earlier, but cause of death was not included until the late nineteenth century.

National statistics leave no doubt that mortality declined rapidly, at least from about 1870. But they also suggest that a significant improvement in health had begun to take place at least a century earlier. This conclusion is based, not on the trend of mortality, which was unknown before 1838, but on the growth of population, to which we must now turn our attention.

The population of England and Wales has been recorded by a decennial census since 1801. There were two earlier estimates, however, one based on a count of families for the Doomsday Book in 1086, and the other on an estimate of the number of hearths in 1695. The growth of population since the eleventh century is shown in figure 1.

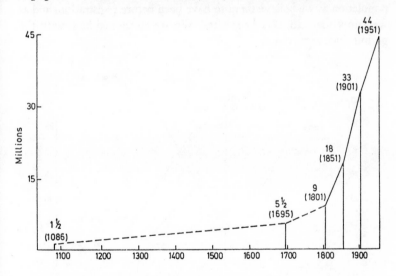

Figure 1. Growth of population of England and Wales.

In the first six centuries the population appears to have rather more than trebled (from $1\frac{1}{2}$ millions in 1086 to $5\frac{1}{2}$ in 1695). It again trebled in the next 150 years (to 1851) and more than doubled in the following 100 years (to 1951). Reasons will be given later for believing that this increase resulted from a decline of mortality and it is the most reliable indication of the period during which health in Britain improved significantly.

Interpretation of the reasons for the improvement presents very different problems before and after registration. After 1838 it is possible to base conclusions on the trend of mortality and on the contribution of different causes of death to its decline. Before 1838 this information is not available, and we must rely mainly on a judgement based on later experience about which we can be reasonably confident. For this reason we shall consider first the change in health since registration.

THE IMPROVEMENT OF HEALTH SINCE REGISTRATION OF BIRTHS AND DEATHS

Figure 2 gives in simplified form the levels of birth rate, death rate and population as we believe them to have been before registration, and as we know them to have been after. We are concerned here with the period since registration.

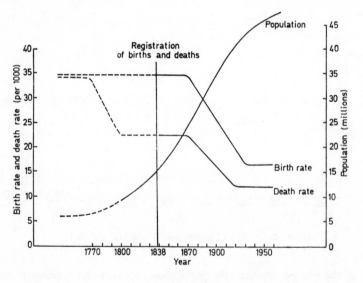

Figure 2. Population, birth rate and death rate: England and Wales.

The figure shows that mortality remained fairly constant between 1838 and 1870 and then began to decline. The continuous growth of population since 1838 is explained by the fact that an excess of births over deaths had been established by that date and has continued ever since. A decline of the birth rate from about 1880 considerably reduced this excess, but because of the further reduction of mortality did not eliminate it.

To explain the continued growth of population it is necessary to account for the reduction of mortality. There is no doubt that it was due almost entirely to a decrease in deaths from infectious disease. This is shown clearly in figure 3, which gives separately the death rates due to infectious and non-infectious causes. The latter undoubtedly include some deaths from infection (such as heart disease caused by rheumatic fever or syphilis) and this probably explains the slight reduction in mortality attributed to non-infectious causes in the nineteenth century.

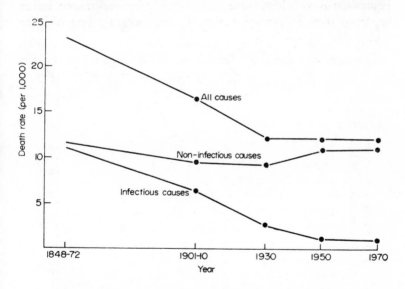

Figure 3. Mean annual death rate (males): England and Wales.

For a closer examination of the diseases which contributed to the decline of mortality we shall consider first the period from 1838 to 1900. Interpretation is more difficult in the twentieth century, when personal medical services were introduced and effective methods of preventing and treating disease in the individual became available (mainly after 1935).

1838–1900

Although cause of death was registered from 1838 it was not treated consistently until the mid century and our examination therefore begins at 1851. Table 2 compares mean annual mortality rates due to certain communicable diseases in the decades 1851–60 and 1891–1900. Five diseases or groups of diseases accounted almost entirely for the decline of mortality in this period: tuberculosis for nearly half; typhus, typhoid and continued fever for about a fifth; scarlet fever for a fifth; cholera, dysentery and diarrhoea for nearly a tenth; and smallpox for a twentieth. The explanation for the reduction of mortality from each of these diseases appears to be as follows.

Tuberculosis

Mortality from tuberculosis was falling in the fifth decade of the nineteenth century, at least thirty years earlier than in the case of the other major infections (figure 4). There is no reliable information about its

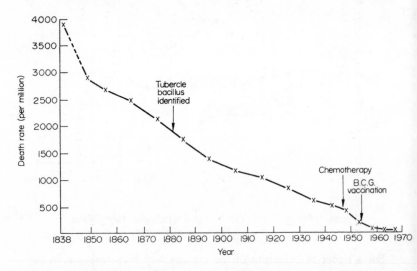

Figure 4. Respiratory tuberculosis—mean annual death rate: England and Wales.

level or trend before registration, although there is no serious doubt that the disease was common in the previous three centuries.

Table 2. Mean annual mortality rates per million living (standardized*) due to certain communicable diseases in decennia 1851-60 and 1891-1900

Cause	1851–60 (a)	1891–1900 (b)	Difference (a)–(b)	Difference per cent of total difference $\frac{(a-b)\ 100}{3,085}$
Tuberculosis—respiratory	2,772	1,418	1,354	43·9 ⎫
Tuberculosis—other forms	706	603	103	3·3 ⎬ 47·2
Typhus, enteric fever, simple continued fever	891	184	707	22·9
Scarlet fever	779	152	627	20·3
Diarrhoea, dysentery, cholera	990	715	275	8·9
Smallpox	202	13	189	6·1
Whooping cough	433	363	70	2·3
Measles	357	398	−41	−1·3
Diphtheria	99	254	−155	−5·0
Other causes	13,980	14,024	−44	−1·4
Total	21,209	18,124	3,085	100

* Standardized to age and sex distribution of 1901 population.

It is useful to consider possible reasons for the decline of mortality from infectious disease under three headings.

1. Medical measures, that is the prevention or treatment of disease in the individual.

2. A 'spontaneous' change in the character of infectious disease, due to a shift in the balance between the virulence of an infective organism and the resistance of the host. The relationship between an infective organism and its host is a changing one, which reflects the influence of nature and nurture on both. However the stability of this relationship differs greatly for different organisms; for example it is much more stable for the tubercle bacillus than for the haemolytic streptococcus.

3. Changes in the environment. Under this heading are included all environmental influences with the exception of medical measures (as defined in 1).

It is clear that medical measures made no contribution to the course of tuberculosis before the twentieth century. In the case of an infectious disease it is never possible to be confident that there has been no change in the balance between the virulence of the organism and the resistance of the host. There appears to have been no significant variation in the tubercle bacillus in the period in which it has been observed. Man's resistance is a more difficult matter; but the fact that the population of Britain had been heavily exposed to the infection for many centuries makes it unlikely that genetic selection was the main reason for the favourable trend in the nineteenth century, since the effect of selection is most evident after first exposure.

Having excluded medical measures confidently and modification of the organism, or of response to it, with reservations (we have concluded only that it is unlikely to have been the most important influence), we are left with changes in the environment as the main reason for the trend of mortality from tuberculosis in the nineteenth century. Four features of the environment need to be considered: conditions of exposure to the disease, diet, and physical and mental stress.

It is unlikely that either physical or mental stress were substantially reduced during the nineteenth century. Exposure to infection is determined mainly by crowding at home or at work; as a result of industrialization and the movement into towns it must have increased in the first half of the nineteenth century and probably did not decrease before its close. By exclusion, admittedly not a wholly satisfactory procedure, we are left with diet as a significant environmental influence.

However the evidence in respect of diet is also positive. The increase in tuberculosis mortality in both World Wars is most reasonably attributed to a deterioration of nutrition. In the nineteenth century, the time when we can be fairly confident that mortality from this disease was declining rapidly—the middle of the century—was also a time when the standard of living was certainly rising. It therefore seems probable that improvement in diet made a significant contribution to the reduction of mortality from tuberculosis during the nineteenth century. This was the conclusion reachèd by Hart and Payling Wright in their study of tuberculosis and social conditions in England.

Typhus, enteric, and simple continued fever

Because they were not separated in national statistics before 1871, these diseases are grouped together. The data are given separately for the last three decades; in this period mortality from enteric fever was reduced by about half and mortality from the other two almost disappeared.

Interpretation of the behaviour of typhus, a louse-borne disease, is complicated by the fact that its prevalence varied greatly at different periods, and it is impossible to say to what extent that was attributable to environmental or genetic change. Nevertheless, it is generally agreed that the disappearance of the disease from the British Isles, many years before identification of the body louse as the vector, was due largely to an improved standard of living. But although a good deal is now known about the nature of the disease and the way in which it is spread, it is still difficult to assess the relative importance of various features of the environment affected by the standard of living. It seems probable, however, that the two main influences were: improved hygienic standards, particularly in respect of water supply and personal cleanliness, which prevented infection by reducing contact with the louse; and better diet, which affected the response to infection. The first of these influences would have begun to operate by about 1880 and the second somewhat earlier.

There is little difficulty in interpretation of the behaviour of typhoid fever. The spread of the disease is due to defective sanitary arrangements, and the rapid reduction of mortality during the last third of the nineteenth century can be attributed confidently to the specific measures, particularly safer water supplies, introduced at that time.

Continued fever still appears in the international classification, where it refers to pyrexias of unknown origin. In the nineteenth century it must have comprised a very mixed group, including undiagnosed respiratory infections such as tuberculosis as well as other fevers in which a rash was either absent or unrecognized. In view of the fact that it was not shown separately before 1871 we can only guess about its earlier behaviour. But since the whole group (typhus, enteric, and continued fever) began to decline sharply in the eighth decade, the most reasonable assumption is that the trend was due to specific hygienic measures which were also responsible for the reduction of mortality from typhus and enteric fever.

Scarlet fever

Views concerning interpretation of the decline of mortality from scarlet fever (figure 5) are probably more consistent than in the case of any other infectious disease. No specific measures of prevention or

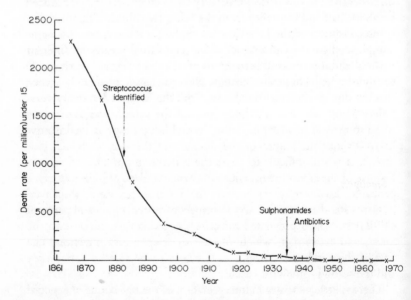

Figure 5. Scarlet fever—mean annual death rate in children under 15: England and Wales.

treatment were available in the nineteenth century, and the only possible explanations are environmental improvement or a change in the nature of the disease. Scarlet fever has exhibited at least four cycles of severity followed by remission. These changes appear to have been largely independent of the environment and there is no reason to differ from the general opinion that they resulted from a modification of the nature of the disease. This is believed to have been due largely to variation in the virulence of the haemolytic streptococcus.

Cholera, dysentery, and diarrhoea

Although these infections were grouped together in national statistics before 1871, cholera must be distinguished from the endemic diseases referred to as diarrhoea and dysentery. Cholera was not endemic in the British Isles, and was introduced from the continent of Europe at least five times during the nineteenth century, but apparently not before. It is therefore not possible to speak of the reasons for its disappearance with quite the same confidence as in the case of the other causes of death.

But with this reservation, there is little doubt about the main reasons for the rapid reduction of mortality from bowel infections in the late nineteenth century. These diseases are spread by infected water and food, and their decline began in the eighth decade when substantial improvements were made in hygienic conditions. There are no grounds for thinking that either therapy or (with a possible reservation in the case of cholera) modification of the nature of the disease made any impact. The reduction of mortality may therefore be attributed to the decline of intestinal infection which resulted from improved hygiene.

Smallpox

Since the contribution of smallpox to the reduction of mortality in this period was small, the reasons for it are less important in the interpretation of the causes of the total decline. This is the disease in which a specific measure—vaccination—appears to have made a substantial contribution, and the only difficulty is to decide how large it was. The fact that smallpox, prevalent for several centuries, declined rapidly from the time when vaccination was introduced suggests that this was an important, and perhaps the main reason for its decline.

Let us now summarize our conclusions. In order of their relative importance the influences responsible for the decline of mortality in the second half of the nineteenth century were (1) a rising standard of living, of which the most significant feature was probably improved diet (responsible mainly for the decline of tuberculosis and less certainly, and to a lesser extent, of typhus), (2) the hygienic changes introduced by sanitary reformers (responsible for the decline of the typhus-typhoid and cholera groups), and (3) a favourable trend in the relationship between infectious agent and human host (which accounted for the decline of mortality from scarlet fever and may have contributed to that from tuberculosis, typhus, and cholera). The effect of specific medical measures was restricted to smallpox and had only a trivial effect on the total reduction of the death rate.

Since 1900

Twentieth century data show that the continued decline of the death rate after 1900 was also due mainly to a decrease in deaths from infectious disease. Between 1901 and 1947 the standardized mortality rate from all causes fell by a half. Nearly a third of this reduction was due to a decrease of mortality from a group of diseases traditionally recognized as 'infectious'. They include the infectious fevers (such as measles, scarlet fever, whooping cough, smallpox and diphtheria), tuberculosis, typhoid, paratyphoid, dysentery, influenza and syphilis. But a further third of the reduction was due to lower mortality from certain groups of diseases which may also be regarded as infectious, since they are caused mainly by pathogenic microorganisms communicable from person to person. These include diarrhoea and enteritis, convulsions in infancy (usually associated with infection) and the respiratory infections, bronchitis and pneumonia. (Although bronchitis in the elderly may in some cases be due primarily to causes other than infections, pathogenic organisms usually contribute significantly to the progress of the disease.)

On this evidence, about two thirds of the reduction in mortality during the first half of the century is attributable to the decline of deaths from infectious disease. Moreover this is probably an underestimate of their contribution, because several other diseases (such as rheumatic heart disease and nephritis) are due primarily to infections.

A most striking feature of the trend of mortality since 1900 has been the decline of infant mortality, that is, of deaths of live born children within the first year of life (figure 6). It was a remarkable feature of the improvement during the second half of the nineteenth century that it had not affected this age group, and at the turn of the century about 150 of every 1,000 children born alive in England and Wales still died within a year of birth. Fifty years later infant mortality was reduced to 30, and it is now less than 20.

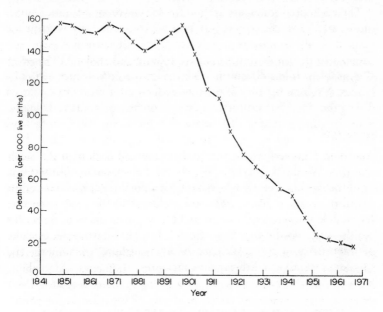

Figure 6. Infant mortality rate: England and Wales.

Assessment of reasons for the decline of infant mortality during the twentieth century (and still more of mortality at all ages), would require a close investigation of different causes of death. Several developments have made this task more complicated than it was in the nineteenth century. In the first place there has been a great extension of medical and related social services. The personal medical services concerned with school health and maternity and child welfare were developed progressively from 1906. The relative importance of the varied measures—cheap and safe infant foods, routine inspection of children, advice about health and treatment—embraced by these services is still uncertain, but there can be little doubt that together they contributed significantly to the saving of infant and child life. In the same period the standard of living continued to rise and was supported by social services. Further advances were made in the control of the physical environment, which had been launched effectively in the second half of the nineteenth century. And, finally, specific measures for preventing and treating disease in the individual began to fulfil the promise of clinical medicine.

There is indeed some justification for the view that without a much more careful investigation it is impossible to express any worthwhile opinion about the relative importance of the influences that have contributed to the improvement in health during the twentieth century. The problem is less difficult if we consider the period since 1838 as a whole. A substantial part of the total reduction of mortality occurred during the nineteenth century, and we are on firm ground in attributing it to the rising standard of living and hygienic measures. Both have continued to advance since 1900, and unquestionably they have contributed powerfully to the further improvement of health since that time. Without denying the value of the personal health services, or of the specific therapy which has been a notable achievement of the past forty years, it seems right to conclude that the main influences responsible for the decline of mortality—our best index of improved health—since deaths were first registered in 1838 have been, in order of importance, a rising standard of living, improved hygiene, and specific preventive and therapeutic measures.

THE IMPROVEMENT OF HEALTH BEFORE REGISTRATION OF BIRTHS AND DEATHS

We must now consider the more difficult problem of interpretation in the period when the national birth rate, death rate and causes of death were unknown. It is one of the ironies of history that the improvement in health appears to have begun at least 70 years before reliable data are available to put the reasons for it beyond dispute. The main evidence of improvement is the fact that the population trebled in size in about a century and a half after 1700, whereas it had risen only from $1\frac{1}{2}$ to $5\frac{1}{2}$ millions in the previous six centuries (figure 1).

From a medical viewpoint it seems reasonable to assume that the increase of population resulted from a decline of mortality. Yet some economic historians suggest that it was due to an increase in the birth rate. They believe that the economic and social changes associated with the Industrial Revolution led to earlier marriage, larger families and a rising birth rate. There is, however, no evidence that there were substantial changes in age at marriage, and at a time when both birth rate and death rate were very high, a decline of mortality seems a more probable consequence of improvements in the environment.

Reasons for the decline of the death rate can be discussed under three headings: medical measures (prevention or treatment of disease in the individual); a 'spontaneous' decline of mortality; and improvement in the environment.

Medical measures

Until recently the decline of mortality in the eighteenth century was believed to be due to medical advances, the explanation proposed by Griffith in his book *Population Problems of the Age of Malthus*. He based this conclusion on medical developments at that time: they included expansion of hospital, dispensary and midwifery services; changes in medical education; and advances in physiology and morbid anatomy.

Serious objections have now been raised to Griffith's interpretation, on the grounds that the medical measures then available are very unlikely to have had a significant effect on national mortality trends. Indeed since they had little influence in the second half of the nineteenth century, it would seem to follow that they were no more effective a hundred years earlier, when knowledge of disease processes was even more incomplete. Nevertheless it has been suggested that there was a measure which might have been important; this was variolation, inoculation by infected material as a protection against smallpox. Although the frequency of variolation is not reliably known, it may have been fairly common, at least in some areas. But to accept that it had a substantial effect on the national death rate we should have to believe that this crude procedure, used without knowledge of its mode of action or full awareness of its dangers, was far more effective than any modern form of immunization. It is not an explanation that appeals to virologists, who consider that variolation is more likely to have spread than to have prevented smallpox. There are therefore no grounds for thinking that medical measures made a significant contribution to reduction of the death rate in the eighteenth century.

A spontaneous decline of mortality

If medical measures are excluded there remain two possible explanations for the eighteenth century reduction of the death rate, a spontaneous decline of mortality from infections and changes in the environment. In the post-registration period, it was possible to identify the diseases which contributed to the decline of mortality and then to consider each disease separately. The same procedure cannot be used before 1838, and we must rely on a judgement of probabilities, assisted by knowledge derived from the nineteenth and twentieth centuries.

The relation between infectious organisms and their hosts is variable, and over any considerable period deaths from some infections would be expected to increase and from others to decrease or remain relatively constant. There is therefore no reason to question that mortality from one or more infections may have declined spontaneously (that is without recognized medical or other intervention) in the eighteenth century, as in the example of scarlet fever at a later period. However the question is whether this explanation can be accepted for the large reduction of mortality and rise of population which occurred before 1838.

Interpretations of this kind have been proposed, particularly with reference to the disappearance of plague. It was suggested that the growth of population in the eighteenth century was analogous to that in two earlier periods when plague declined and disappeared, the first from the mid eleventh to the late thirteenth century and the second from the mid fifteenth to the end of the sixteenth century. On this interpretation the eighteenth century rise of population was not considered unique, except in having started from a higher level and maintained its momentum for a longer period.

There are several reasons for rejecting this explanation. In the first place, the causes of death before the nineteenth century are not reliably known, and conclusions based on the behaviour of individual diseases are largely speculative. And secondly, it is extremely unlikely that the substantial decline of mortality which must have occurred in the eighteenth and early nineteenth centuries was due wholly or even predominantly to the behaviour of a single disease.

But there is an even more serious objection to attributing the decrease of the death rate and growth of population before 1838 to a spontaneous decline of infectious diseases. The eighteenth century expansion was the beginning of the modern rise of population which has continued to the present day. In duration, continuity and extent, as well as in its relation to the Agricultural and Industrial Revolutions it was a unique phenomenon and requires a unique explanation. It cannot be considered analogous to earlier and transient increases of population, which may be attributed plausibly to the ebb and flow of mortality from infectious disease. We conclude therefore that while spontaneous fluctuation of deaths from infections may have influenced the death rate over short periods in the eighteenth century, it cannot have contributed substantially to the large decline of mortality and growth of population which occurred between 1700 and 1838.

Improvement in the environment

The conclusion that neither specific medical measures nor a spontaneous decline of infectious diseases accounts for the decline of mortality and expansion of population in the eighteenth and early nineteenth centuries makes it necessary to consider the third possibility, that there was a significant improvement in the environment. We can be fairly confident that it was not in hygienic conditions, which deteriorated with industrialization and the growth of towns in the nineteenth century, and can hardly have improved substantially before the passing of the 1848 Public Health Act, and probably not before the eighth decade (when mortality from intestinal infections began to decline).

There is however an important feature of the environment in respect of which there is impressive evidence of improvement, namely food supplies. Food production in England and Wales increased greatly during the eighteenth and nineteenth centuries; it was sufficient, at times more than sufficient, to feed the rapidly expanding population and it was not until the later part of this period that it was supplemented significantly by imported food. This improvement resulted from advances in agriculture which spread throughout Europe from the end of the seventeenth century. Initially these changes were not of a technological kind; they comprised essentially an extension of traditional methods such as conservation of fertility, enclosure, crop rotation, winter feeding and extension of land under cultivation. These measures, with the introduction of root crops and improved transport, brought about a change from exploitive to productive agriculture, and it was not until the nineteenth century that they were supported to any extent by chemical and other technological methods.

The conclusion that an increase in food supplies was the main reason for the decline of mortality and growth of population before the mid nineteenth century rests on three considerations: first, that the other possible explanations are found unacceptable; second, that there was undoubtedly a great increase in home grown food; and third, that in the circumstances which existed prior to the Agricultural Revolution, an improvement in food supplies was a necessary condition for a substantial and prolonged expansion of population. The last point is based on the belief that prior to the eighteenth century the growth of population was restricted mainly by a high level of mortality attributable to insufficient food. This is essentially the Malthusian interpretation and we see no reason for not accepting it.

REASONS FOR IMPROVEMENT IN HEALTH

It is now possible to bring together our conclusions concerning the modern improvement in health. It began in the eighteenth century and was reflected in a decline of mortality which has continued, with interruptions, until the present time. The improvement was initiated by an increase in food supplies which resulted from the Agricultural Revolution that spread throughout Europe after 1700. From about 1870 this influence was powerfully supported by improved hygiene, particularly in respect of water supplies and sewage disposal. And in the twentieth century, further advance followed the introduction of effective preventive and therapeutic measures, mainly after 1935, the year when the sulphonamides were first used.

Together these influences were responsible for a rapid expansion of population, brought about by the increase in life expectation which resulted from improvement in human health. But in time, and on an evolutionary scale a fairly short time, the advance in health would have been reversed, as other advances during man's history were reversed, by expanding numbers, if birth rates had not also declined. In England and Wales for example, if the birth rate had remained at its eighteenth century level, the population today would be nearly three times as great, with profound consequences for welfare and health. From a historical viewpoint, therefore, the limitation of population growth by control of family size was an indispensable condition for improvement, without which all other influences would in time have become ineffective.

This interpretation of the modern advance in health and rise and eventual control of population puts the emphasis on the following: increased food supplies from the early eighteenth century; limitation of numbers and removal of adverse influences in the environment by improved hygiene from the late nineteenth century; and specific medical measures (immunization and therapy) from the second quarter of the twentieth century. The contribution of the last influence to the total decline of mortality was relatively small and the improvement in human health therefore was due predominantly to a change in reproductive behaviour and to modification of the environment by provision of food and protection from physical hazards. It should also be noted that only two of the four major influences were introduced in order to improve health; the reasons for increasing food supplies and limiting numbers were only indirectly related to this objective.

But while the contribution of specific medical measures attributable to medical science and technology was relatively small, the contribution of science and technology as a whole was large. So far as can be judged, the initial and very considerable increase in food supplies in the eighteenth century owed little to science and technology, since the agricultural changes which led to them were neither chemical nor mechanical, and in countries such as Ireland and Sweden occurred long before industrialization. But from the nineteenth century the improvements were advanced further by scientific agriculture and by the rising standard of living which resulted from the Industrial Revolution. Similarly, while it is unlikely that scientific methods played any considerable part in birth control in the late nineteenth and early twentieth centuries, the advances in understanding which led people to limit the size of their families were closely related to the rising standard of living. And finally, although hygienic measures were introduced without knowledge of microorganisms, the control of communicable disease was greatly extended by the developments in microbiology which followed the work of Pasteur.

Hence, while the major influences responsible for the modern improvement in health were not due initially to science and technology, they were all subsequently indebted to science. Science extended the relatively simple methods which led to the first advances in agriculture, in hygiene and in birth control. It also provided a basis of understanding which ensured that the advances were not lost, as others (for example Roman hygiene) had been lost at earlier periods of man's history.

FURTHER READING

BURNET M. (1953) *Natural History of Infectious Disease*. Cambridge University Press, Cambridge.

CREIGHTON, C. (1965) *A History of Epidemics in Britain*. Frank Cass & Co. Ltd., London.

D'ARCY HART P. and PAYLING WRIGHT G. (1939) *Tuberculosis and Social Conditions in England*. National Association for the Prevention of Tuberculosis, London.

GLASS D. V. and EVERSLEY, D. E. C. (eds.) (1965) *Population in History*. Edward Arnold Ltd., London.

GREENWOOD M. (1935) *Epidemics and Crowd Diseases*. Williams and Norgate, London.

GRIFFITH G. T. (1967) *Population Problems of the Age of Malthus*, 2nd Edition. Frank Cass & Co. Ltd., London.

MCKEOWN T., BROWN R. G. and RECORD R. G. (1972) 'An Interpretation of the Modern Rise of Population in Europe', *Population Studies*. **XXVII,** 345.

MALTHUS T. R. (1960) *Essay on the Principle of Population*. Everyman's Library, J. M. Dent & Sons Ltd., London.

2 · EFFECT OF THE DECLINE OF THE DEATH RATE ON MEDICAL PROBLEMS

CONSEQUENCES OF IMPROVED HEALTH

Introduction

Since the time of Kepler and Harvey medical thought has been dominated by the belief that improvements in health must rely largely on an engineering approach, based on understanding of the structure and function of the body and of the disease processes which affect it. This approach was based on a physical model, in which a living organism was conceived as a machine which might be taken apart and reassembled if its structure and function were fully understood. In medicine this concept led to the belief that an understanding of disease processes and of the body's response to them would make it possible to intervene therapeutically, mainly by physical (surgical), chemical or electrical methods.

The consequences of this conceptualization of the medical task are even more conspicuous in medicine today than they were in the seventeenth century, largely because the resources of the physical and chemical sciences are so much greater. Medical education begins with the study of the structure and function of the body, continues with examination of disease processes and ends with clinical instruction on selected sick people; medical service is dominated by the image of the acute hospital where the technological resources are concentrated; and medical science reflects the mechanistic concept, for example in the attention given to the molecular basis of inheritance and the immuno-logical response to transplanted organs. Indeed the question is not whether the engineering approach is predominant in medicine, which would hardly be disputed, but whether it is deficient as a conceptualization of the problems of human health.

Our examination in Chapter 1 of reasons for past improvement in health suggest that the traditional conceptualization is in fact deficient, at least in relation to the changes of the past two centuries. We concluded that the major contributions to the improvement were from limitation of family size (a behavioural change), an increase in food supplies and a healthier physical environment (environmental influences). The contribution of specific preventive and therapeutic measures is recent and relatively limited.

This conclusion is in accord with experience of requirements for the health of living things other than man. In domestication of animals, their numbers and distribution are controlled; they are provided with more and better food; and they are protected so far as possible from environmental hazards, including parasites, predators and extremes of weather. Hence improvements in livestock, like improvements in the health of man, have resulted primarily from measures directed to populations rather than to individuals.

However, in technologically advanced countries the advances of the past two centuries have inevitably had a profound effect on the character of medical problems and it is conceivable that the major influences on health may no longer be the same. The common causes of sickness, disability and death have changed, primarily in response to the influences considered in Chapter 1, but also as a secondary consequence of a different age distribution of the population.

Changes in causes of sickness and death

The predominant influence has been the decline of mortality from infectious disease; some diseases are now much less common (tuberculosis and typhoid) while others have virtually disappeared (smallpox and cholera). This decline has made certain other conditions relatively more prominent (congenital malformations) although their incidence may be no greater than in the past.

The effects of the reduction of deaths from infections have been profound, and it is questionable whether we shall ever again see a change in the spectrum of disease and disability as great as that which has occurred in the past century. Indeed the twentieth century may come to be recognized as a watershed, separating the infectious diseases which were formerly predominant from the residual problems when infections are reduced to small proportions. Changes in these residual problems are of course inevitable, but they are likely to be small in comparison with those which have already occurred.

The change in age distribution

The age distribution of the populations of developed countries has changed in response to two influences, the trend of mortality within

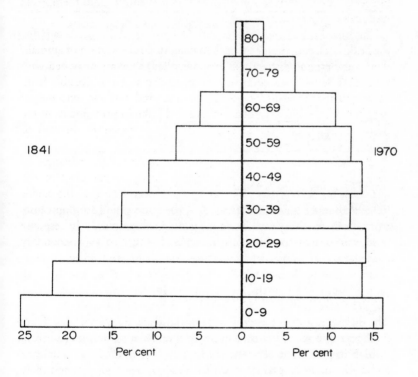

Figure 7. Age distribution of the population of England and Wales in 1841 and 1970.

age groups and, to a lesser extent, the decline of the birth rate. Figure 7 compares the age distribution of the population of England and Wales in 1970 with that in 1841.

(a) *The trend of mortality within age groups*

Since deaths from infectious disease were most common in early life. the trend of mortality during the past century has been different at different ages. In 1970 the death rate was 52·4 per cent of that in 1841–50 (table 3). The reduction was very great in early life, substantial in middle life and moderate in late life.

Table 3. Change in death rates between 1841–50 and 1970 (England and Wales)

Age	1970 rate as percentage of 1841–50 rate
0	11·9
1–14	2·7
15–44	9·5
45–64	47·0
65 and over	68·4
All ages	52·4

(b) *The decline of the birth rate*

The birth rate has declined (from 35·5 per 1,000 population in 1871–75 to 16·0 in 1970), and at first sight it might appear that this influence also would have contributed to the higher age of the present day population. However it is the change in the number of births rather than in the birth rate which affects age distribution, and since the annual number of births is approximately the same in England and Wales today as in 1870, it is unlikely to have had much influence on the difference in the age distributions shown in figure 7.

Figure 8 shows the change in the relation between mortality and age which has occurred between 1838–54 and 1970. It gives the number of deaths per 1,000 conceptions for five age periods: prenatal, 0–14, 15–44, 45–64 and 65 and over. Mortality after birth was estimated by applying to the numbers liveborn (estimated below as 770 per 1,000 conceptions in both 1838–54 and 1970) data provided in English life tables for the relevant years. The only uncertainties are about prenatal losses which are based on the figures shown in table 4.

Contemporary estimates of the proportion of conceptions aborted spontaneously appear to be reasonably reliable and are about 140 per

1,000; there is no reason to believe that this figure has changed greatly since the mid nineteenth century.

The frequency of legal abortions has risen rapidly since the liberalization of the grounds for abortion in 1968 and the figure for 1970 (70 per 1,000) is based on the number of legal abortions reported in that year.

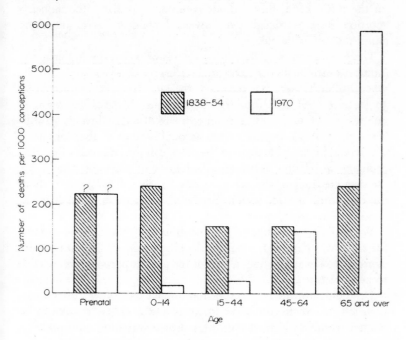

Figure 8. Mortality (per 1,000 conceptions) at different ages.

Table 4. Estimates of prenatal deaths in 1838–54 and 1970

	Deaths per 1,000 conceptions	
	1838–54	1970
Spontaneous abortions	140	140
Legal abortions	Nil	70
Illegal abortions	50	10
Stillbirths	40	10
Total	230	230

The estimates of illegal abortions are the least reliable, since even today their number is unknown. But it seems probable that in view of the recent change in the law the number of pregnancies terminated illegally is now small, and it has been assumed to be 10 per 1,000. The figure shown for 1838–54 (50 per 1,000) can be no more than a guess; on the one hand it seems certain that it was higher than it is today; on the other hand, the methods commonly available for inducing abortion were restricted and unwanted children were sometimes eliminated by infanticide.

The proportion of stillbirths for 1970 is based on the stillbirth rate (number of stillbirths per 1,000 total births) for that year. For 1838–54, when stillbirths were not recorded, the rate has been assumed to be 50 per 1,000 total births (stillbirths plus livebirths); the earliest recorded rate was 40 in 1928. This gives an estimate of approximately 40 stillbirths per 1,000 conceptions when account is taken of abortions.

It would be desirable to assess the change in the character of medical problems in relation to sickness, disability and premature death. But the data are limited, and we must rely largely on information about cause of death, making such inferences about morbidity and disability as seem permissible.

We shall first assess the relation of mortality to age. From national life tables it is possible to estimate the proportions of liveborn persons expected to die at stated ages, but for the present purpose it is desirable to begin at conception.

On these estimates, the proportion of conceptions which terminate prenatally is of the order of 20 to 25 per cent. So far as can be judged from the limited data, this proportion does not appear to have altered substantially since the mid nineteenth century. However, since the changes in the abortion law in 1968 there has been a rapid increase in legal abortions and, almost certainly, a decrease in illegal abortions.

Figure 8 shows the remarkable change in the age distribution of deaths that has taken place during the past century. The notable features are: (a) little change in prenatal deaths (in spite of the decline of the stillbirth rate, for the contribution of this to the total of prenatal losses is not large); a reduction in the number of deaths in early and middle life, marked at ages 0–14 and 15–44 and small at 45–64; and an increase in deaths at 65 and over. This increase is due, not to a rise in death rates, but to the increased number of people surviving to late life.

PROBLEMS AT DIFFERENT AGES

Birth to age 14

The very large reduction of mortality in the prereproductive age group since 1838–54 (figure 8 and table 3) is attributable predominantly to a decline in deaths from infectious disease. This decline has occurred throughout childhood, but was most marked in the first year of life when mortality was formerly greatest (figure 6). The infant mortality rate (number of deaths under 1 year per thousand liveborn children) fell from 150 in 1901 to 18 in 1970.

The decline of infections has increased the relative importance of some other causes of death which in the same period have shown little or no improvement; it has also altered the balance between deaths due to prenatal and postnatal causes. Table 5 gives for 1970 death rates by cause of death for stillbirths, deaths in the first week after birth and deaths in the remainder of the first year. Two points should be noted: first, that more than half of infant deaths now occur within a week of birth; and second, that the common causes of stillbirths and early postnatal deaths are the same. The last feature has led to the introduction of the perinatal death rate—the number of stillbirths and deaths in the first week after birth expressed per 1,000 total births. Perinatal deaths are due to influences operating before (mainly) or during birth, and their increased frequency relative to infectious deaths in infancy is among the most striking changes which have resulted from the decline of mortality from infectious disease. In 1970, infections—mainly bronchitis and pneumonia—were responsible for less than a quarter of all infant deaths.

Table 6 analyses deaths between the end of the first year and age 14. In this period mortality is low and the most common causes of death—formerly the infections—are now accidents and violence and neoplasms. It should be noted that table 6 gives annual death rates per 1,000 living; that is to say it gives the risk of dying in a single year for all those in the age group. For an individual aged 1 year the risks of death before the fifteenth birthday would be roughly fourteen times greater than those estimated in table 6.

Our conclusions concerning mortality between conception and age 14 can be summarized as follows. There are approximately 250 deaths per 1,000 conceptions in this age period, of which about 220 are

Table 5. Death rates (per 1,000 live and stillbirths) by cause (England and Wales 1970)

Cause of death	Stillbirths	Deaths in first week after birth	Deaths in remainder of first year
Complications of pregnancy and birth			
Toxaemia of pregnancy	1·20 ⎫	0·09 ⎫	— ⎫
Difficult labour	0·72 ⎬ 7·69	1·08 ⎬ 2·29	0·07 ⎫
Conditions of placenta and umbilical cord	4·45 ⎪	0·23 ⎪	0·01 ⎬ 0·10
Other specified complications of pregnancy and birth	1·32 ⎭	0·89 ⎭	0·02 ⎭
Congenital malformations	2·52	1·71	1·95
Infections			
Acute respiratory infection, bronchitis, pneumonia	—	0·25 ⎫ 0·29	2·92 ⎫ 3·71
Other infective conditions	—	0·04 ⎭	0·79 ⎭
Neoplasms	—	—	0·08
Accidents and violence	—	0·05	0·58
Other specified conditions	0·61	0·90	0·72
Ill-defined and unknown causes	2·19	5·18	0·33
All causes	13·02	10·43	7·47

Table 6. Annual death rates (per 1,000 living) from principal causes (England and Wales 1970)

Age 1–14

Accidents and violence	0·14
Neoplasms	0·07
Congenital malformations	0·06
Respiratory infections	0·06
Other infectious diseases	0·04
Other causes	0·07
All causes	**0·44**

Age 15–44

Accidents and violence	0·33	
Neoplasms	0·28	
Ischaemic heart disease	0·13	⎫
Cerebrovascular disease	0·05	⎬ 0·25
Other circulatory diseases	0·08	⎭
Respiratory infections	0·07	
Other infectious diseases	0·02	
Other causes	0·16	
All causes	**1·11**	

Age 45–64

Ischaemic heart disease	2·88	⎫
Cerebrovascular disease	0·87	⎬ 4·61
Other circulatory diseases	0·86	⎭
Neoplasms	3·41	
Respiratory infections	1·05	
Other infectious diseases	0·09	
Accidents and violence	0·44	
Other causes	0·79	
All causes	**10·39**	

Age 65 and over

Ischaemic heart disease	16·12	⎫
Cerebrovascular disease	10·67	⎬ 36·33
Other circulatory diseases	9·54	⎭
Neoplasms	11·05	
Respiratory infections	10·50	
Other infectious diseases	0·24	
Accidents and violence	1·45	
Other causes	5·12	
All causes	**64·69**	

abortions, 10 are stillbirths and 20 deaths between birth and age 14. Of the latter, about 9 occur within the first week after delivery.

To complete assessment of the medical problems in the prenatal and prereproductive periods we must consider handicaps and sickness in childhood. There are no means of assessing fully the extent of either of these problems but numbers of children in special schools provide an indication of the frequency of severe handicap. In England and Wales approximately 11 per 1,000 school children are so handicapped that they require admission to special schools. The commonest types of handicap are educational subnormality (which accounts for more than half of the total), limitations of sight and hearing and a variety of other physical abnormalities due to conditions such as congenital malformations, cerebral palsy and infectious disease. Handicaps due to infections are now much less common than formerly; but there is no evidence of a significant reduction in the incidence of congenital handicaps such as mental subnormality, which now account for a large majority of those affected. But the prevalence of these conditions in the population has increased because the proportion of handicapped people who survive to maturity and even to late ages is today much greater than formerly, chiefly as a result of an improved standard of living and better hygiene, rather than because of direct medical intervention. It follows that the problems of congenital handicap are no longer mainly restricted to childhood; indeed the majority of those living with the commonest abnormality—mental subnormality—are adults.

It is even more difficult to assess accurately the frequency and causes of sickness in childhood. A lower demand for paediatric hospital beds suggests that there has been a reduction of morbidity from infections in parallel with the decline of mortality. Nevertheless infectious disease in childhood remains a considerable problem and is the most common reason for consulting a general practitioner about the health of children. There are also large problems associated with non-fatal accidents and violence. However, a considerable part of the problem of sickness, particularly serious sickness, like the problems of handicap and death, has been determined by the time of birth, and is associated with causes such as malformations, immaturity and birth trauma.

Apart from the reference to mental subnormality, this discussion of problems in early life has been restricted to physical causes of mortality and disability. Problems of mental illness also present in all age groups, but since they can be considered more meaningfully together, they will be discussed at the end of this section.

Ages 15-44

Mortality in the age group 15-44 has fallen sharply and is now about one-tenth of the level in 1841-50 (table 3). As in the younger age group, the improvement has been due to a reduction of deaths from infectious disease. A hundred years ago tuberculosis was the most common cause of death and infections were responsible for most of the mortality. Today the common causes of death are accidents and violence, neoplasms and cardiovascular disease (table 6). Together these causes account for three-quarters of the total mortality while infectious diseases are responsible for only about one-tenth.

Since ages 15-44 represent approximately the reproductive age group we must refer briefly to death of women in childbirth. From the beginning of this century maternal mortality remained fairly constant until 1934, since when it has declined from 4·6 deaths per 1,000 total births to 0·18 in 1970. This change was due largely to the control of puerperal infections by chemotherapy and the effective use of blood transfusion. Nevertheless there is little doubt that a considerable proportion of the maternal deaths that remain—a recent investigation suggested about two-fifths—are potentially avoidable.

Ages 45-64

Between 1841-50 and 1970 mortality at ages 45-64 declined by about half (table 3). This again is accounted for mainly by the behaviour of the infections: in 1848-72 the death rate attributed to the specified infectious diseases (of which the most common were tuberculosis and pneumonia) was 8·0 (of a total death rate of 22·3 per 1,000); in 1970 it was 1·1 (of a total of 10·4). Because of the vagaries of the earlier classification it is difficult to interpret the trends of other causes of death, but cancer appears to have increased in frequency and cerebral haemorrhage and accidents to have decreased.

The common causes of death at ages 45-64 are now those shown in table 6. In order of frequency they are cardiovascular disease (including cerebrovascular disease), neoplasms, respiratory infections (especially bronchitis) and accidents and violence. In this age group the so-called degenerative diseases have become predominant, for the order of frequency of causes of death is the same as at ages 65 and over.

It is again difficult to assess fully the extent of sickness and disability. Before age 65, indeed before 69, the disabilities commonly associated with ageing—defects of hearing, vision, mobility, etc.—are relatively uncommon. The usual causes of short term sickness and disability are accidents, respiratory infection and rheumatism; and of prolonged disability they are bronchitis, mental illness and arthritis.

Ages 65 and over

Figure 8 suggests that about two-thirds of individuals conceived now die after 65. For those aged 65 and over, mortality has declined since 1841–50 by about a third (table 3). In this age group, because of the unsatisfactory earlier classification of causes of death, it is difficult to speak confidently about reasons for this change. (What should perhaps be noted at this point is that the relation between the decrease in death rates shown in table 3 and the increase in expectation of life over the same period is deceptive. For example, between 1838–54 and 1970 expectation of life of males increased by 12·5 years at age 15, 4·4 at age 45 and 1·2 at age 65. These increases are smaller than might have been expected in view of the substantial reduction of mortality in the corresponding age groups.)

The common causes of death at 65 and over (table 6) are the same as in the previous age group: cardiovascular disease, neoplasms, respiratory infections and accidents and violence. The common illnesses which bring patients to general practitioners are respiratory disease (especially chronic bronchitis), arthritis and rheumatism, accidents and cardiovascular disease. From age 69 the frequency of physical and mental disabilities increases rapidly and a large proportion of hospital beds is occupied by the aged who are either physically or mentally ill.

Mental illness

Assessment of the problems associated with mental illness encounters the familiar difficulties of recording accurately and meaningfully conditions which cause sickness and disability rather than death. There are no data which make it possible to examine experience of mental illness over a prolonged period, and for recent years conclusions must be based mainly on the results of special investigations, and on the useful observations on patients in psychiatric hospitals in England and Wales, published by H.M.S.O. since 1953.

With due regard for the limited evidence, there are two conclusions concerning the trend of mental illness which are not in doubt. The first is that with one important exception, the pattern of mental illness has not been modified by the decline of infectious disease to anything like the same extent as the pattern of physical illness, for the obvious reason that most psychiatric disorders are not of infective origin. The exception is in the case of syphilis affecting the central nervous system; once a common cause of admission to psychiatric hospitals, it has now virtually disappeared.

The second trend which is evident is an increase in the proportion of psychiatric patients at older ages. To a considerable extent this is explained by the changed age structure of the population as a whole; since mental illness is more common in old than in young people, its age distribution must change in an ageing population. But it is also probable that the improvement in expectation of life during the past century has been greater for psychiatric patients, as for other handicapped groups such as the mentally subnormal, than for the population as a whole (because, when conditions for survival are unfavourable, as they were until recently, the survival of the handicapped is likely to be more affected than that of the rest of the population).

From the limited evidence it is difficult to be confident about the trend of the total volume of psychiatric illness. The data for psychiatric hospitals in England and Wales show that between 1954 and 1969 (a) the number of in-patients per 1,000 population fell by 31 per cent, (b) the proportion of long stay patients in hospital for two years or more decreased from 76 per cent to 65 per cent and (c) the number of admissions (of which nearly half were readmissions) increased by 150 per cent. The explanation of these trends will be considered more fully later in relation to psychiatric services, but here it may be said that more active treatment is increasing the frequency of admission to hospital while reducing the size of the hospital population. The net effect of the multiple influences—changing age structure of the population, more active treatment and changes in economic, social and other conditions—on psychiatric problems as a whole is unknown.

THE CHARACTER OF CONTEMPORARY HEALTH PROBLEMS

In assessing the character of the residual health problems of technologically advanced countries it is important to distinguish between genetic and other diseases. The term genetic disease is properly used in reference to conditions due to disorders of genes or to recognizable abnormalities of chromosomes. All other diseases and disabilities, while influenced by various degrees of genetic predisposition, are not attributable to any identified genic or chromosomal disorder, and whether and when they are manifested is determined largely by the environment to which the individual is exposed.

Prenatal life

Natural selection has restricted to a low frequency conditions due to disorders of genes, whether manifested before, at or after birth. A much larger number are attributable to abnormalities of chromosomes arising mainly at fertilization, but most of these are eliminated as spontaneous abortions. Hence most prenatal deaths and congenital abnormalities (those present at birth, whether recognized or unrecognized) are due to the hazards associated with implantation and embryonic and fetal development. In a few cases these hazards come from outside the uterus, as in the examples of malformations caused by thalidomide and rubella; but in most they are determined by intrauterine conditions which are far less susceptible to control. It is therefore not surprising that in a period when there has been a large reduction of postnatal mortality, there has been only a modest decrease in stillbirth rates, and apparently no change in the annual incidence of congenital malformations or mental subnormality. For although prenatal deaths and congenital disabilities are susceptible to the influence of natural selection, the environmental conditions which lead to them are relatively constant and difficult to control.

Prereproductive and reproductive life

In assessment of the character of the residual health problems these two periods may be considered together. Since natural selection has restricted the frequency of conditions due to disorders of genes, and most of these due to chromosomal abnormalities are eliminated before birth, the proportion of individuals affected at birth or later by genetic disease is small, probably well below 1 per cent. The large majority of diseases and disabilities presenting in the prereproductive and reproductive periods are therefore due to environmental influences, operating before birth in the case of congenital conditions and after birth in the case of abnormalities determined postnatally.

Postnatal influences are much more accessible than those which are prenatal, and as noted in Chapter 1, improvement in health has been due largely to their control—by provision of more food and removal of hazards from the physical environment. However even in the most advanced countries the control of such hazards is far from complete. Moreover a new class of environmental risks has been added, the self-imposed risks of smoking, excessive or unbalanced diet and deficient exercise. These influences will be considered more fully in Chapter 10, but here it should be noted that they already play an important part in determining the health problems in the reproductive and postreproductive periods.

Postreproductive life

In conditions manifested after the end of reproduction the effects of natural selection are reduced or absent. Hence while the frequency of genetic disease and disability due to disorders of genes or chromosomes is very low, genotypes causing a strong predisposition to abnormality are relatively more common in late life than at lower ages. Nevertheless there is no reason to doubt that a considerable proportion of the diseases presenting in the postreproductive period are due to environmental influences which may have operated over many years, even as early as childhood. These influences include both the general environmental hazards (deficient food, atmospheric pollution, accidents, etc.) and the self-imposed risks such as smoking and lack of exercise.

ETHICAL ISSUES ASSOCIATED WITH CONTEMPORARY HEALTH PROBLEMS

The advances of the past two centuries have resulted in a considerable extension of life for handicapped as well as for normal people. To a large extent this prolongation is due to general influences such as better food and hygiene which no humane society would wish to withhold; but it has also become possible to extend by treatment the lives of patients who are permanently disabled, and this raises the general issue of the ethics of medical intervention in such cases. The issue is most discussed in relation to the elderly, but it arises even more poignantly in respect of those who are severely handicapped from birth and may survive for many years as a result of treatment.

The discussion which follows will be based on congenitally malformed children who epitomize the extent and nature of the problem of medicated survival.

About three in every hundred children are born with recognizable physical abnormalities, which may vary from a trivial blemish of the skin to a serious condition of the heart or brain. Most of these malformations raise no large medical or ethical issues, either because they present no threat to the quality or duration of life, or because they are so lethal that effective medical intervention is almost inconceivable. The proportion of malformed children whose lives can be substantially prolonged by treatment is certainly not more than 1 in 6 and probably less than 1 in 10.

Against this background the problem of the malformed raises three issues: prevention by contraception; elimination by abortion; and treatment from birth. Within that part of the future which it is realistic to discuss, it seems very unlikely that the conception of malformations will be preventable to any appreciable extent by genetic engineering or by recognition of parents likely to give birth to an affected child. Identification of the seriously malformed embryo or fetus early in pregnancy is now occasionally possible. It may become more so, in which case abortion would probably be regarded by most, though not all, doctors as the procedure of choice. But now and in the immediate future, the problem of the malformed is essentially the problem as it presents from birth.

There is no dispute concerning the treatment of most malformed children. No one is likely to question the desirability of closing a cleft palate, or of surgery in congenital heart disease where operation offers the prospect of normal life to patients who would die early if untreated. The problem arises where the outcome of treatment is the survival of a child with a serious physical or mental handicap, and this occurs particularly in relation to the malformations of the central nervous system.

In such cases the desirability of treatment must be examined with two considerations in view: the quality of life which is prolonged by medical intervention; and the price paid in care of the handicapped, particularly by close relatives, but also by the community at large through provision of social, educational and medical services.

It is at this point that controversy begins and it is important to distinguish between those whose principles allow no account to be taken of quality of life or cost of care—they hold that life should be

prolonged wherever possible without regard for the consequences—
and those whose conscience allows no such escape from the dilemma
presented by some of the most serious malformations. This distinction
can be illustrated by reference to the abnormality of anencephalus,
characterized by gross maldevelopment of the brain and death before
or within a few hours of birth. Logically, anyone who thinks that no
account should be taken of the consequences, should agree that it
would be a proper goal of medical research and practice to provide
a vegetable existence for the anencephalic, without regard for the cost
to public services and the distress of close relatives, particularly the
parents. But those who cannot accept this extreme interpretation of
humanism must face the formidable problem of deciding in respect of
other malformed births with what degree of handicap and at what
price to the community they would consider it undesirable to intervene to prolong life.

In relation to these issues, the malformation of spina bifida is something of a test case. The condition is the result of failure of the spinal
cord to close during prenatal development. By closing the lesion the
surgeon is able to prolong the lives of children who without treatment
would die soon after birth. Some of these children will be paralyzed
and incontinent for the rest of their lives, and some will be mentally
retarded as well. Moreover, most of those who are paralyzed are
known to be irreversibly paralyzed from birth.

Since the patient cannot represent himself, and a careful weighing
of the complex medical, ethical and other issues is almost impossible
for the distraught parents, the decision in such cases must usually be
taken by the obstetrician, paediatrician or neurosurgeon. Unless he
takes the uncompromising view that all lives must be saved, the doctor
has to decide whether to intervene in relation to the criteria referred
to above: the quality of the life prolonged; and the cost of survival
to the community.

As judged by the number of places needed in special schools, the
cost to the community of surgical intervention in all operable cases
of spina bifida would be very great, and in time, no doubt, medical
decisions will have to be influenced by considerations of this kind.
These judgements will be most difficult when something like a normal
life can be achieved at very high cost. In the case of spina bifida,
however, the issue is simplified by the fact that what is achieved at
high cost is often not a normal life but a cruelly handicapped one. A
life indeed of such quality that many doctors think it wrong to

prolong it even if no price were paid by the community in supportive services.

This raises what is perhaps the central problem posed by the treatment of congenital deformities, and indeed of the seriously handicapped in general: on what basis can a judgement be made that the quality of life will be such that it should not be prolonged? There is no other test than this: would I wish myself to live, or to have my own child survive from birth with such a handicap? When confronted by the prospect of lifelong paralysis from spina bifida, some doctors have no doubt about their answer.

FURTHER READING

BURNET M. (1971) *Genes, Dreams and Realities*. Medical and Technical Publishing Co. Ltd., Aylesbury, Bucks.

DUBOS R. (1959) *Mirage of Health*. George Allen and Unwin Ltd., London.

DUBOS R. (1968) *Man, Medicine, and Environment*. Pall Mall Press Ltd., London.

McLACHLAN G. (ed.) (1972) *Patient, Doctor, Society: A Symposium of Introspections*. Oxford University Press for the Nuffield Provincial Hospitals Trust, London.

Symposium: The Cost of Life, *Proc. roy. Soc. Med. Lond.* **60** (1967), 1195–1246.

Symposium on Ethics in Medical Progress. Ciba Foundation, J. & A. Churchill Ltd., London (1966).

3 · EFFECT OF THE DECLINE OF THE BIRTH RATE AND DEATH RATE ON THE GENETIC CONSTITUTION OF THE POPULATION

In this chapter we shall consider whether the improvements in health of the past two centuries have been achieved at the price of an increase in the proportion of genetically handicapped individuals. This is a complex issue on which opinion is sharply divided. Some people believe that genetic equilibrium is being seriously disturbed, and that unless appropriate eugenic measures are taken genetic deterioration is inevitable. Others consider that such fears are exaggerated, and that in any case the measures suggested are for one reason or another likely to be unacceptable or ineffective. Although these differences of opinion are not wholly of scientific origin, the fact that experienced observers have arrived at quite different conclusions reflects both the complexity of the problem and the inconclusive nature of much of the evidence.

The belief that genetic equilibrium is being disturbed is derived from two considerations. First, because of the improvement in health, many people who formerly would have died at an early age now survive and reproduce. Some of them pass to their children genes associated with disease and disability. This, it is suggested, must increase the frequency of harmful genes. Second, measured intelligence is consistently a little higher in school children from small than from large families. This has been interpreted to mean that conception is controlled more rigorously by the intelligent than by the less intelligent, and it is concluded that this too must have had an undesirable effect on the genetic constitution of the population.

Among objections which have been raised to these interpretations two are so fundamental that if they are accepted there is little need for further discussion. We shall therefore examine them at the outset.

1. The conclusion about the consequences of improved survival has been criticized on the grounds that a gene which is undesirable in one environment is not necessarily so in another. For example genes which are harmful in wild animals may be advantageous after domestication, since fitness must be redefined in relation to the new environment. Similarly, it is suggested, changes in gene equilibrium which result from modification of man's environment are not necessarily undesirable.

However, this objection does not take account of the complexity of the problem in man. If an increase in gene frequency is a secondary consequence of a more or less permanent change in the character of the environment, for example of a shift from rural to urban life, or improvement in diet, no ill-effects need be anticipated so long as the change is maintained. The fact that the population of Western Europe is probably more susceptible to cholera and typhoid now than in the mid nineteenth century may not matter because the source of infection is effectively controlled. The circumstances are quite different if increased gene frequency is a direct result of medical therapy; for a disease such as diabetes, which is compatible with survival and reproduction, may have unpleasant features for those afflicted. Moreover, the services required to care for affected people are to some extent provided at the expense of alternative uses of medical effort.

2. The negative correlation between fertility and intelligence is also said to be misinterpreted. A similar correlation exists between fertility and other variables such as stature and longevity which show no evidence of a decline. (Indeed both have been increasing.) In the *Biology of Mental Defect*, Penrose gives reasons for thinking that in such cases differential fertility may be a natural biological process, consistent with genetical equilibrium. The same explanation has been suggested for the differential birth rate with respect to intelligence.

However, while genetic stability is consistent with differential fertility, there is no reason to doubt that it can be disturbed by selective restrictions in breeding. Extreme variation of weight and length have been produced in farm animals by selective breeding, and it is possible that the differential use of contraception has influenced human intelligence.

Hence we conclude that if improved health has increased the frequency of genes associated with disease, to the extent that this has raised the incidence of diseases which are unpleasant or require medical treatment it must be regarded as undesirable. And if the negative correlation between intelligence and sibship size does not permit us to conclude that intelligence is declining, the concept of genetic stability does not dismiss the possibility. Thus we cannot on *a priori* grounds accept the view that a change in the genetic constitution of human populations could not have occurred, or that such a change would be unimportant. Both suggestions result from pressing the analogy with animal populations without sufficient regard for the unique circumstances associated with the growth of the population since the eighteenth century. In the first place, although the reduction of the death rate was attributable largely to environmental changes which might be regarded as analogous to domestication, to the extent that it was due to medical therapy it can be described fairly as unique. And secondly, the introduction of effective measures of birth control may have superimposed on the pattern of natural fertility a new pattern not determined primarily by the activity of the ovary and the testis. It is at least possible that this change has had some genetic significance. Certainly it would have social significance, for even if no genetic influence were involved, we could not regard it as unimportant if family limitation were practised most intensively by those who could create the most favourable environment for their children.

THE EFFECT OF THE DECLINE OF MORTALITY

It would be easier to assess the possibility that improvements in health are disturbing genetic equilibrium if we could be more confident about the mechanisms which maintain it. On the face of it, genes which prejudice survival or fertility should in time be eliminated; and in view of the length of man's history it may be asked why a condition such as haemophilia still exists. It is due to a sex linked recessive gene, which is constantly being destroyed because the fertility of those affected is low. Yet the incidence of haemophilia appears to remain fairly constant at about 1 per 15,000 of population. Two possible explanations are known.

Genes lost may be replaced by mutation. The mutation rates in man which have been estimated are low, but they are enough to affect substantially the frequency of rare conditions, such as haemophilia and achondroplasia.

A second explanation for the persistence of harmful genes is the phenomenon of heterosis. It is best known in plants, whose hybrids commonly exhibit vigour which may be absent or less conspicuous in the pure strains. Evidence of the same kind is available in animals, including man.

The basis of heterosis can be illustrated by reference to a condition such as sickle cell anaemia. Those affected (the homozygotes) have a pair of genes associated with an abnormal type of haemoglobin. But unaffected individuals with the unpaired abnormal gene (the heterozygotes) appear to have a selective advantage (possibly through being more resistant to malaria) over both homozygotes and normal individuals without the gene. Thus the reduction of genes from the loss of homozygotes may be offset by the increase from the improved survival of heterozygotes.

But although mechanisms of this kind tend to maintain genetic stability, there can be little doubt that the improvement in health since the eighteenth century has raised the frequency of some genes related to disease. For the increased expectation of life has been due mainly, until the present century wholly, to a decline of mortality from infectious disease. In the past, in order to reproduce, an individual had to survive and remain fertile after extensive early exposure to a wide range of infections. This must have been among the most powerful influences in natural selection, and its substantial reduction in technologically advanced countries has undoubtedly produced a population genetically less fit with respect to certain infections. But whether this change should be regarded as undesirable depends on the nature of the influences which have brought it about. In Chapter I it was concluded that they were as follows.

Improvement in diet

This was considered to be the most important influence on the decline of mortality and growth of population in the eighteenth and early nineteenth centuries. It was probably the main reason for the decline of tuberculosis, and the population may be genetically more susceptible to this disease now than formerly. But whether this is undesirable depends upon the possibility of a reversal of the conditions under which the susceptible have survived and reproduced. Specifically, since improved diet and a rising standard of living have been the most significant influences the question is whether they are likely ever again to be reduced. It is ironic that in a nuclear age an unequivocal answer cannot be given, but it is perhaps not unduly optimistic to regard the improved living standard as a permanent feature in countries where it has been achieved. If this is so, the modification of the genetic constitution of the population which has resulted may not be unfavourable.

Better hygiene

Hygiene was judged in importance to be second only to food supplies. It is probable that the population is now genetically more susceptible to cholera, typhoid and other intestinal infections, and the question is again whether the means responsible for this change are permanent. It seems reasonable to believe they are, for the methods which ensure a clean water supply (for example) are not costly and are specific in their effects on disease. Hence in a developed country there is little reason to be concerned about increased susceptibility to diseases which are preventable by hygienic measures.

Spontaneous change in the character of disease

Scarlet fever and influenza are outstanding examples of diseases whose behaviour appears to have been essentially independent of both medical measures and environmental changes, and to be due to modification of the relationship between the infective organism and the host. Mortality from both diseases has varied greatly during the present century, and the genetic susceptibility of the population may also be presumed to have varied. But this variation appears to be independent of human intervention and is a cause rather than a consequence of improved health.

Specific medical measures

In the nineteenth century smallpox was the only disease significantly affected by specific measures and their contribution to the total decline of mortality from infections to the present time has been smaller than that of other influences. It is hardly possible to predict the long term consequences of immunization on genetic susceptibility to infectious disease. Since many people have survived and reproduced who formerly would have died in childhood it is certainly possible that the number of susceptibles has increased. But vaccination and immunization procedures provide substantial protection which may compensate for any genetic change which has resulted from them. Treatment has been relatively less important, and is unlikely to have had much effect on the genetic basis of susceptibility.

Broadly, if infectious disease can be prevented, provided the measures are inherent in changing living conditions, or (if they are not inherent) are not too costly, an increase in the incidence of susceptibles is probably of little consequence. In the case of most infections from which mortality has declined during the past two centuries these conditions have been met. At the same time it must be admitted that long term predictions are hazardous, unless the source of infection is effectively controlled. It is conceivable that an organism such as the tubercle bacillus may adapt by mutation to the unfavourable conditions now offered by the human body.

The probabilities for non-infectious diseases are somewhat different. Some have responded to the same environmental influences which led to the decline of infections and the significance of genetic change is similar. For example, an increase in the proportion of children who require a higher level of nutrition might be unimportant, because the improved diet can probably be maintained. But an increase in the frequency of disease which is unpleasant or requires continued therapy would certainly be undesirable.

There is little evidence that therapy has so far altered the frequencies of genes associated with disease or disability. In a common condition such as diabetes, where the effect of treatment on survival and reproduction has been striking, the genetic basis of the disease is obscure. And in the few uncommon conditions, such as haemophilia and fibrocystic disease of the pancreas, where the genetic background is fairly clear, the increase in life expectations has as yet had little effect on reproduction.

THE EFFECT OF CONTRACEPTION

Although the birth rate in England and Wales undoubtedly fluctuated in earlier centuries as a result of changes of mortality, and possibly in relation to other influences such as age at marriage, it was not until the late nineteenth century that it began to show the effect of intentional restriction of family size. There is little evidence of birth control in the English demographic literature of the seventeenth century, and it is doubtful whether abstinence has had much influence on population growth.

The observation that measured intelligence is a little higher in children from small than from large families suggests that contraception may have altered the pattern of differential fertility. Whether it has done so is not clear. The negative correlation between intelligence and sibship size might be wholly due to biological causes; but we cannot exclude the possibility that to some extent it also reflects the influence of contraception. No conclusion about the trend of intelligence can be drawn from the fact that other variables such as stature, also negatively correlated with sibship size, have not decreased. For the only question which arises in the present context is whether family size has been more restricted by the intelligent than by the less intelligent. If contraceptive practice is associated with stature it would be as a secondary consequence of its correlation with intelligence.

Since the evidence is inconclusive we must try to give a common-sense answer. And common sense suggests that it is likely that intelligent people made early and efficient use of contraceptives, as they must have made early and efficient use of other amenities provided by the sanitary revolution.

However, the interpretation of this conclusion is complicated by the fact that to an unknown extent intelligence reflected in both test performance and reproductive behaviour is environmentally determined. The higher scores by children from small families, or the greater use of contraceptives by intelligent parents, might be due to their favourable environments rather than to their superior genes. If this is so the restricted reproduction may have little or no influence on the transmission of genes which determine intelligence.

The available evidence gives no answer to the very theoretical question whether, in a uniform environment in which contraceptives were readily available, variation in fertility in relation to intelligence would be greater than could be attributed to biological influences alone. But it seems reasonable to suppose that it would, since the level of intelligence below which people are incapable of practising contraception is probably higher than the level below which they are invariably infertile. That is to say there are fertile individuals of low intelligence who are incapable of limiting the size of their families. Their frequency is unknown, and the effect of their reproduction on the pattern of differential fertility would be determined to some extent by the practice of other fertile people. In a society in which small families have considerable advantages, those with the ability to limit family size will do so, and the influence of the larger families of fertile individuals of low intelligence would be greater than in a society in which the penalties for large families were less severe.

For these reasons it seems possible that the spread of contraceptive knowledge has had some influence on the trend of the intelligence which is measured by tests, and a smaller and perhaps trivial influence on the genetic component in intelligence. This conclusion is based, not on the negative correlation between measured intelligence and sibship size, which might be largely due to biological variation, but on consideration of the extent to which contraception may have been practised by individuals of varying intelligence.

Finally let us consider whether if such a trend exists it is of any practical importance. It seems to be widely believed that a general increase in intelligence would be highly desirable, and that even a small decline, particularly of the genetic component in intelligence, would be a serious matter which would require urgent action. This opinion overlooks the fact that there exists an immense reserve of unused ability which is more accurately assessed in Gray's *Elegy in a Country Churchyard* (a poetic expression of the nature nurture viewpoint) than in some discussions of the trend of intelligence. Unless we are prepared to believe that there have been some remarkable mutations at different times in history, we must conclude that it is only in certain places and for very short periods that any considerable part of the capacity available has been exploited.

FURTHER READING

HOGBEN L. (1945) *Nature and Nurture*. George Allen and Unwin Ltd., London.
PENROSE L. S. (1963) *The Biology of Mental Defect*, 3rd Edition. Sedgwick & Jackson, London.

4 · THE MEASUREMENT OF ILL HEALTH

Before health priorities can be determined and health resources deployed to the best advantage it is necessary to know what the major disease problems are. Until recently deaths were the only source of information about the pattern of ill health in Britain.

MEASUREMENT OF MORTALITY

Number of deaths and age at death have been reliably recorded for more than a century; reporting of cause of death is less reliable. The tabulations of deaths by cause published each year by the Registrar General are an analysis of what different generations of doctors with varied medical backgrounds have written on death certificates. They represent an analysis of opinions rather than facts, for fashions in diagnosis change and as knowledge advances nomenclature of disease also changes. For example, when death registration was introduced in 1838, fewer than 100 causes of death were distinguished and these included as major categories 'want of breast milk', 'convulsions', 'privation', 'diarrhoea' and 'old age'; today the current International Statistical Classification of Diseases, Injuries and Causes of Death (I.C.D.) lists more than 1,000 diagnostic entities.

In Chapter 2 the principal causes of death in England and Wales were discussed in some detail. Table 7 reminds us that about one quarter of all deaths in this country are now attributed to ischaemic heart disease and one fifth to cancer. Next in order of magnitude come

cerebro-vascular disease, other heart conditions, bronchitis and
emphysema and, a long way behind, accidents. But the crude death rate
(the number of deaths per 1,000 total population) provides a very
incomplete and, indeed, a misleading picture of the amount of serious
disease in the population. For, other things being equal, the more old
people there are in a population, the higher the crude death rate will
be: the crude death rate is lower in Birmingham than Bournemouth
and in Ebbw Vale than Llandudno, not because Birmingham and
Ebbw Vale are healthier but because Bournemouth and Llandudno
are places to which many elderly people move after retirement. Deaths
in infancy, childhood and young adult life represent a much more

Table 7. Leading causes of death in England and Wales 1970 (males and
females of all ages)

I.C.D. No.	Cause of death	No. of deaths	Death rate per 1,000 population	Percentage distribution
410–414	Ischaemic heart disease	139,317	2·8	24·2
140–209	Malignant neoplasm	115,729	2·4	20·1
430–438	Cerebrovascular disease	79,291	1·6	13·8
393–404 } 420–429	Other heart conditions	46,733	1·2	8·1
490–493	Bronchitis, emphysema and asthma	30,181	0·6	5·3
800–999	Accidents, poisonings and violence	22,701	0·5	3·9
	All other causes	141,242	2·6	24·6
	All causes	575,194	11·7	100·0

serious loss to the community than deaths in old age. There are many
ways of making allowance for age at death in comparing different
populations. One is to consider only age specific death rates, for
example the stillbirth rate (number of stillbirths per 1,000 total live
and stillbirths registered in a year), the infant mortality rate (deaths of
infants under one year per 1,000 live births registered) or death rates
for five-yearly age groups (i.e. 0–4, 5–9, 10–14, etc.). There are also
various ways of standardizing death rates for age and of calculating
standardized mortality ratios (the S.M.R. gives an age adjusted death rate

converted to a percentage of the death rate in a standard population).

However, even when age is taken into account and the cause of death given on the death certificate is reasonably reliable (as it now is in Britain), only when there is a high case fatality rate (number of deaths per hundred cases of the disease) does the death rate provide any measure of the frequency with which a disease occurs. For example, in 1970 cancer of the respiratory system (I.C.D. 160–163) was responsible for 25,841 male and 5,657 female deaths; in the same year the deaths of 5 males and 3 females were attributed to neuroses (I.C.D. 300). The first number provides a good measure of how common cancer of the lung is (more than 90 per cent of all cases die within five years of diagnosis); the second gives no indication of the size of the problem presented by the neuroses.

If deaths are a poor indication of the amount of disease in a community, they are an even more inadequate measure of the suffering, disablement, inefficiency and loss of working time caused by ill-health. In national mortality data a death from an immediately fatal road accident is given the same weight as a death at the same age from mitral stenosis preceded by many years of impaired health, a major and costly operation and a period of extreme disablement. In short, therefore, although in the nineteenth century death rates forcibly demonstrated that at that time the over-riding disease problem was one of epidemic and endemic infectious disease, today, when infection is a much less common cause of death and mortality in infancy and young adult life is very much lower, more refined measures of the amount and distribution of ill-health are required. We need to know how often, for how long and from what causes people are ill as well as the rate at which they die.

MEASUREMENT OF MORBIDITY

In addition to innumerable ad hoc surveys, there are now many routine sources of information about the amount of ill-health in the community. Some of the more important sources are given in table 8.

For many reasons measurement of ill-health is more complex than measurement of mortality. There is no clear line between health and sickness as there is between life and death; death is a unique event which takes place at a point in time, whereas illnesses have a duration, can recur and have different degrees of severity.

Table 8. Sources of information about morbidity

1. Notification of Disease and Disability

(a) Notification of Infectious Disease
(b) Notification of Industrial Disease
(c) Notification of Congenital Malformations (recorded at Notification of Birth)

2. Registration of Disease and Disability

(a) Blind Persons' Register
(b) Disabled Persons' Register
(c) Cancer Register

3. National Health Service Records

(a) Hospital Records
(b) General Practitioner Records
(c) Health Visitor and Child Welfare Clinic Records
(d) Home Nursing Records

4. School Health Service Records

(a) Routine Examinations
(b) Special Schools' Records

5. National Insurance Records

(a) Sickness Claims
(b) Industrial Injuries Claims

6. Industrial Health Service Records

(a) Sickness Absence and Accident Records of Large Firms
(b) Examination of Persons engaged in certain Dangerous Processes

It has been pointed out that there is a zone between sickness and health in which the decision whether a person is sick depends on definitions of health and the individual making the judgement. If a man believes he is ill, he is suffering from something, if only a delusion, and in that sense he is sick even if his doctor is unable to find a physical explanation. On examination for life insurance, or as a result of a screening procedure, a man who believes he is healthy may be found to have a disease which soon will cause disability or death (e.g. chronic nephritis, or carcinoma of the lung). Clearly, although he is not conscious of ill-health, in a very real sense he is ill. The science of bacteriology first drew attention to this type of difficulty by uncovering the carrier state, and the development of biochemical, haematological and other laboratory tests have underlined it by presenting the clinician and epidemiologist with comparable problems in the field of non-infectious disease (for example diabetes, anaemia, cancer of the cervix, hypertension).

Difficulties also arise because illnesses have a duration and because over a given period the same person may suffer from more than one illness. Many different indices of morbidity are therefore possible. For example, in a defined population we can count all the illnesses present at a point in time (point prevalence), all the illnesses present at any time during a defined period (period prevalence), or illnesses that begin during a defined period (incidence). In the same way instead of illnesses we can count persons who are ill. (The same person may have more than one cause of ill-health at a given time, or may suffer from more than one illness, or may develop the same illness more than once, over a defined period.) These complications have given rise to a great deal of terminological confusion, so that in any statement about morbidity it is essential to define the index used.

Finally, measurement of the severity of illness presents its own problems. Indices such as time off work, confined to house or bed, out-patient attendance, admission to hospital and duration of stay in hospital all have their uses and limitations.

It should now be clear that there can be no precise answer to the question: how much ill-health is there in the population. Indeed if we accept the definition of health provided by the World Health Organization—'a state of complete physical, mental and social well being and not merely the absence of disease or infirmity'—we are all sick. But if definitions of ill-health are used which are less all embracing and more precise, answers of considerable medical interest can be provided. It is useful to look at the problem at four different but not altogether mutually exclusive levels: ill-health most frequently complained of; ill-health leading to general practitioner consultation; ill-health causing absence from work; and ill-health leading to hospital admission.

Illnesses most frequently complained of

A continuous survey of sickness in the population of England and Wales was carried out by the Central Office of Information from 1943 until 1952. The data were collected by direct interview, not from records of patients using the medical services, with the intention of assessing, among other things, the amount of ill-health which did not come to medical attention. Each month men and women in representative samples of the adult population were interviewed by non-medical field workers about the illnesses they had experienced during the previous three months. The definition of illness was broad and included anything the individual considered to be a disturbance of his health during the period.

Table 9. Illnesses most frequently complained of (Survey of Sickness, 1949)

Nature of Illness	Number of Illnesses	Percentage of Total
Rheumatism	16,133	12·1
Digestive disorders	14,642	10·9
Colds, Influenza	14,115	10·6
Other Respiratory Illnesses	9,642	7·2
Eye Affections	6,370	4·8
Dental disorders	5,289	4·0
All other illnesses	67,129	50·4
Total	133,320	100·0%

There are obvious weaknesses in morbidity statistics based on what a person remembers and is prepared to tell a non-medical interviewer about recent ill-health; nevertheless they provide useful information that cannot be obtained in any other way. Two out of three persons reported an awareness of some ill-health during the month before the interview, and, as expected, awareness of ill-health increased steeply with age. Less expected was the finding that at all ages females complained of more ill-health than males. In spite of the very high proportion of the population reporting awareness of ill-health, only one in four of those complaining had seen a doctor and only one in eight had lost time from work or been confined to the house during the month. Rheumatism, digestive disorders and colds, influenza and other respiratory conditions were the illnesses most frequently reported (table 9). This type of survey draws attention to the fact that there is a great deal of minor and ill-defined illness in the population which causes little incapacity and rarely leads to consultation with a doctor.

Illnesses for which people consult general practitioners

Much useful information about sickness in the population is stored in general practitioners' records. A large enquiry involving 170 doctors in 100 practices in different parts of England and Wales was carried out by the College of General Practitioners in collaboration with the General Register Office for the twelve months beginning May, 1955.

Table 10. Leading causes of general practitioner consultations

Nature of Illness	Number of Consultations	Percentage of all Consultations
Acute and chronic bronchitis	92,995	6·2
Acute Nasopharyngitis	62,501	4·2
Influenza	40,668	2·7
Acute tonsillitis	34,136	2·3
Benign hypertension	31,136	2·1
Anxiety reactions	28,819	1·9
All other conditions	1,211,697	80·7
Total	1,501,952*	100·0%

* 50,172 routine maternity consultations have been excluded.

In table 10 the illnesses for which people most often consult their doctors are given. Although there is much minor ill-health for which medical advice is not sought, about two thirds of all patients on a doctor's list consult him either in their own homes or in his surgery at least once during a year; and over the same period he gives an average of four consultations per patient on his list. Much the commonest reasons for consultation are upper and lower respiratory diseases, followed by raised blood pressure and anxiety reactions. This pattern of ill-health is not unlike that reported by people in morbidity surveys but is very different from that displayed by mortality statistics (table 7). Indeed, coronary disease and cancer, responsible for more than one third of the deaths in the country, do not appear among the first ten reasons for practitioner consultation.

Illnesses which cause absence from work

Medical certificates of incapacity for work are required by the Department of Health and Social Security to support claims to sickness or injury benefit. Analysis of the claims provides information of great administrative importance, and on the face of it should also be a valuable source of data about morbidity in the population. From this point

Table 11. Leading causes of absence from work, Great Britain 1968

Diagnostic Group	Millions of days lost	Percentage distribution
Bronchitis	38·58	11·8
Mental, psychoneurotic and personality disorders	30·68	9·4
Accidents, poisonings and violence	27·00	8·2
Diseases of digestive system	26·40	8·0
Other diseases of respiratory system	25·40	7·8
Arthritis and rheumatism	23·98	7·0
All other conditions	156·44	47·8
Total	327·58	100·0

of view, however, the data have to be interpreted with caution. In the first place, the whole population is not covered, for many women and some men are not gainfully employed. Second, much minor illness is excluded, for spells of incapacity of less than four days are not normally subject to benefit. Third, duration of absence is not a very reliable measure of the severity of an illness. A man's attitude to his work, his employer's and fellow workers' attitude to him, the security of his job, the loss of income involved (whether he is also entitled to benefit from private insurance, works sick club, etc.) and many other factors may affect the period of absence. Finally, the reason given on the medical certificate for sickness absence is imprecise and sometimes unreliable or even misleading, for the general practitioner knows that his certificate will be seen by the patient and by a number of lay persons, including possibly the patient's employer. Hence the diagnosis he enters is often purposely indeterminate. With these reservations the most important cause of absence from work among the insured population is bronchitis, which accounts for about one in eight of all days lost (table 11). Also of great importance are mental conditions, accidents, digestive disorders, other diseases of the respiratory system and arthritis and rheumatism—again a very different pattern from that displayed by mortality, but recognizably related to general practitioner consultations.

Illnesses treated in hospital

Since hospitals are the most costly segment of the medical services, a regular flow of information about use, staffing and cost of hospital

Table 12. Leading diagnoses for discharges and deaths from non-psychiatric hospitals, England and Wales 1970

Diagnosis	Number of discharges and deaths	Percentage distribution
Fractures, dislocations and other injuries	505,860	12·8
Diseases of digestive system	492,510	12·4
Diseases of respiratory system	463,400	11·7
Cardiovascular diseases	459,130	11·6
Malignant and benign neoplasms	378,360	9·6
Diseases of breast and female genital system	253,610	6·4
All other conditions	1,405,040	35·5
All conditions	3,957,910*	100·0

* Excludes 949,830 conditions of pregnancy, childbirth and puerperium.

beds is important administratively. Case records also provide a useful index of the amount of serious illness in the population. Hospitals send to the General Register Office for analysis detailed information about one in ten of all out-going patients. No other source of morbidity statistics provides data about diagnosis with so much detail and reliability, but the sample of illnesses is highly selected. Nearly every case of some conditions (such as perforated peptic ulcer) is admitted to hospital. But for many others, the decision whether to admit or to treat at home is influenced by social class, domestic circumstances, availability of beds, interests of general practitioners and other factors which vary from area to area and time to time and are only loosely related to severity of illness. The analysis of reasons for hospital treatment (table 12) reveals a pattern of disease greatly influenced by the need for surgery. This is the pattern medical students see during their clinical years and it bears little resemblance to the pattern of ill-health reported by the general population or seen by general practitioners.

5 · MORTALITY AND MORBIDITY IN BRITAIN TODAY

The decline of mortality in Britain which began in the eighteenth century has continued to the present time. Death rates from nearly all causes have been falling, but a few major diseases have shown increases that warrant the description of epidemics. Moreover it is not surprising that it is possible to identify subgroups of the population which differ widely in experience of disease, since there are large differences in living standards and medical services are by no means uniformly adequate.

MODERN EPIDEMICS

During the past 50 years, for both males and females, there have been increases in the frequency of ischaemic heart disease and cancer of the lung of epidemic proportion. Because of changes in the International Classification of Diseases, the ageing of the population and advances in diagnostic precision, it is difficult to get reliable data about the magnitude of the increase over the whole period. However, death rates in the years 1960–70 were not greatly affected by these influences and they show that the epidemics are continuing (table 13). During the decade, death rates (per million) for ischaemic heart disease increased by 16 per cent for males and 14 per cent for females and for cancer of the lung by 23 per cent for males and 63 per cent for females. It should be mentioned that, when corrected for the change in the age structure of the population over the decade, these percentage increases

Table 13. Modern epidemics in England and Wales (certain causes of death for which death rates are increasing)

I.C.D. No.	Cause of death	Males		
		Death rates per million		Percentage increase
		1960	1970	1960–70
410–414	Ischaemic heart disease	2,927	3,392	16
162	Malignant neoplasm of bronchus lung and trachea	852	1,045	23

I.C.D. No.	Cause of death	Females		
		Death rates per million		Percentage increase
		1960	1970	1960–1970
410–414	Ischaemic heart disease	2,032	2,324	14
162	Malignant neoplasm of bronchus lung and trachea	131	214	63
174	Malignant neoplasm of breast	382	424	11
183	Malignant neoplasm of ovary	124	144	16

are a little reduced. Although these two epidemics are known to be due largely to personal habits (cigarette smoking, unsatisfactory diet and lack of physical exercise: see Chapter 10), it has not yet been possible to control such influences. At every age death rates for most causes are lower for females than for males, but death rates for cancer of the lung are increasing more steeply for females than for males (as is the amount they smoke). Deaths attributed to cancer of the breast and cancer of the ovary are also increasing, for reasons which are not yet clear.

REGIONAL DIFFERENCES IN DISEASE INCIDENCE

When death registration was made compulsory in 1838 it was immediately obvious that there were striking regional differences in death rates. Broadly speaking the death rates increased with latitude and to a lesser extent this is still true today—death rates tend to be lowest in the south and the east and highest in the north and the west.

This pattern is well illustrated by the stillbirth and infant mortality rates for 1970 (table 14). The trend is due in part to recognizable differences in living conditions; the young infant is very sensitive to adverse environmental influences. Death from infectious disease or accident may result from a low standard of maternal care, over-crowding, malnutrition and bad housing (often associated with inade-quate facilities for washing, cooking and food storage; defective sanitation; and unsatisfactory arrangements for room heating and refuse disposal). There is less overcrowding in the south than in the

Table 14. Stillbirth and infant mortality rates by region (England and Wales 1970)

Region	Rates per 1,000 total births		Rates per 1,000 live births
	Stillbirths plus infant deaths	Stillbirths	Infant deaths
East Anglia	27·0	11·2	15·9
South East (including London)	27·8	11·5	16·4
South West	28·5	11·7	16·9
East Midlands	30·1	12·8	17·6
North (including Tyneside)	32·4	14·0	18·7
West Midlands (including Birmingham conurbation)	32·9	14·3	18·9
Wales	33·2	14·8	18·7
Yorkshire and Humberside	34·2	13·9	20·6
North West (including Manchester and Liverpool conurbations)	35·7	15·0	21·0

Midlands and north of England, which have a legacy of congested and insanitary working class housing from the nineteenth century. Wales and Scotland have always been less prosperous than England and were particularly hard hit during the difficult years between the two world wars.

As would be expected the regional difference is greatest for the postneonatal period (from the beginning of the second to the end of the twelfth month of life). Pneumonia, gastroenteritis and bronchitis still make a substantial contribution to the death rate during that period, and mortality from these diseases is greatly influenced by adverse living conditions. That perinatal mortality (stillbirths and deaths during the first week of life per thousand total births) should also show a regional pattern is less expected, for the leading causes of death are of natal and prenatal origin (congenital malformation, immaturity, birth injury). Many influences are involved: for example, standards and availability of health service vary from area to area, and even within the limited range of latitude of England and Wales climate may play a part in determining regional differences. Climate certainly influences the regional pattern of mortality from respiratory infections and chronic bronchitis, which is much the same as that for infant mortality. Evidence is also accumulating that the death rate from ischaemic heart disease, which follows a similar pattern, is related to climate (low temperature and high humidity).

Two striking regional differences in disease incidence for which as yet there are no convincing explanations should also be mentioned. Death rates for cancer of the stomach are more than 30 per cent higher in Wales than in England, and the incidence of neural tube defects (anencephalus and spina bifida) in South Wales is among the highest in the world. The malformations of the central nervous system are particularly common in the mining communities of Glamorgan and Monmouthshire.

URBANIZATION AND DISEASE

When related to the size of the urban community in which they occur, death rates are highest in the so-called conurbations and decrease through large and medium sized towns to their lowest level in small towns and rural areas. This association of death with city dwelling is almost all due to an increase of death rates from respiratory diseases with increasing size of town (table 15). People living in and near large cities are subject to very much higher death rates from bronchitis, cancer of the lung, respiratory tuberculosis and pneumonia than those living in the country. Death rates from most other conditions, including ischaemic heart disease and cerebrovascular disease (together now responsible for 38 per cent of all deaths), bear little or no relation to size of town. Exposure to the irritants poured into the atmosphere of cities from coal consumed in domestic grates and in the ovens and furnaces of industry is the likely explanation for much

Table 15. Standardized Mortality Ratios* of males (England and Wales = 100) for certain causes of death related to size of town (1970)

I.C.D. No.	Cause of Death	Conurbations	Large Towns	Medium Towns	Small Towns	Rural Areas
				Size of Town		
490–492	Bronchitis, emphysema	118	107	100	98	74
162	Cancer of lung and bronchus	119	106	99	90	78
010–012	Respiratory Tuberculosis	134	109	96	78	69
480–486	Pneumonia	117	107	100	88	85
410–414	Ischaemic Heart Disease	103	103	99	104	91
430–438	Cerebrovascular Disease	96	99	102	105	100

* The S.M.R. is the ratio per cent of the observed number of deaths in a given population divided by the number of deaths which would have occurred if the age-specific mortality rates for England and Wales had applied in that population.

of this difference (see Chapter 16). It may also be due to the increased risk for city and town dwellers of contracting airborne infection when travelling to or at work, and in places of entertainment. In the past this played an important part in the spread of respiratory tuberculosis.

For many medical and most surgical conditions hospital admission rates are also higher for town than for country dwellers and are highest for those living in the conurbations. The reason is not clear. Utilization of health services is determined as much by the facilities available as by the need for them, and whether admission rates for such conditions as uterine fibromyoma, haemorrhoids, tonsillar hypertrophy and hernia are much higher in conurbations than in rural districts because these conditions are commoner among city dwellers or because there is a greater awareness of the need for treatment and a much readier access to hospital services in the cities is a matter for investigation.

OCCUPATION AND DISEASE

An industrial society presents a wide range of occupational environments and patterns of work which may affect health. In Chapter 18

Table 16. Occupational mortality for males aged 45–54 at the census of 1851 (after William Farr)

Occupation	Mortality per 1,000 living
Farmer	11·1
Shoemaker	15·0
Weaver	15·4
Grocer	16·5
Blacksmith	16·5
Carpenter	16·7
Tailor	16·7
Labourer	17·3
Miner	20·1
Baker	21·2
Butcher	23·1
Innkeeper	28·3
All males	17·9

the implications of this fact are discussed in relation to control of disease. Here we shall consider briefly occupational mortality at national level.

Information about occupation is obtained from relatives at death registration and occupation is recorded for the whole population at each census. At or near the census years, therefore, deaths can be related to the working populations in which they have occurred to give occupational mortality rates. William Farr made the first official study of this type. Using data from the census of 1851, he calculated mortality rates for males in several hundred different occupations. For the age group 45–54 he found that farmers had the lowest and innkeepers the highest mortality (table 16).

For various reasons data such as these are difficult to interpret. First, mortality in many occupations is influenced by the type of men recruited into them. For example, jobs making heavy physical demands tend to attract the fitter and more active members of the working population, while men with respiratory tuberculosis, cardiovascular disease and chronic bronchitis often seek jobs which make light physical demands. Second, mortality in hazardous occupations, such as coalmining and foundry work, is understated because workers

Table 17. Some occupations with high and low S.M.R.'s for all causes. Males aged 15–64 (England and Wales 1959–63)

High Ratios	S.M.R.
Deck and engine room ratings, barge and boatmen	193
Coal mine face-workers	180
Stage managers, actors, entertainers, musicians	148
Publicans, innkeepers	147
Fishermen	144
Constructional engineers and riggers	142
Low Ratios	
University teachers	56
Other teachers	60
Clergy, ministers, members of religious orders	62
Dental practitioners	64
Farmers, farm managers, market gardeners	72
Electrical and electronic fitters	78
Medical practitioners	89

whose health has been seriously undermined by such employment may transfer to less exacting occupations and these are recorded at death registration. Third, information about occupation given by relatives is not always reliable; the relative may not know the job of the deceased, or may upgrade it. Finally, a difficulty arises from the different age structures of persons in different occupations. To take an extreme example, there would be little point in comparing mortality of medical students with that of senior physicians. Allowance is made for the last difficulty in the standardized mortality ratio. The S.M.R. has many uses. For example, different occupations can be compared in respect of all causes of death taken together. Table 17 shows that at the time of the 1961 census, deck and engine room ratings and coal mine face workers were subject to death rates nearly twice the national average and four times the death rates of university and other teachers. Mortality among registered medical practitioners was 89 per cent of the national average.

Table 18. Some occupations with high and low S.M.R.'s for cirrhosis of liver. Males aged 15–64 (England and Wales 1959–63)

High Ratios	S.M.R.
Publicans and innkeepers	773
Stage managers, actors, entertainers, musicians	550
Deck engineering officers and pilots	467
Cooks	460
Lodging house, hotel keepers, housekeepers and stewards	450
Low Ratios	
Shop salesmen and assistants (non-food)	38
Teachers	44
Drivers, motormen, fireman (railway engines)	50
Machine tool setters, setter operators	50
Drivers of buses, conductors	64

Occupations can also be compared in relation to a specific cause of death. Table 18 shows, not unexpectedly, that publicans and inn-keepers have a mortality from cirrhosis of the liver eight times the national average and sixteen times that of teachers.

Mortality from specific causes of death in a particular occupation can also be compared with the national average. Table 19 suggests that doctors have a much higher than average mortality from cirrhosis

Table 19. Some disease specific S.M.R.'s for male medical practitioners under 65 years of age

I.C.D. No.	Cause of Death	S.M.R.
581	Cirrhosis of liver	350
E963, 970–979	Suicide	176
420	Coronary disease, angina	118
330–334	Vascular lesions of CNS	110
140–205	Malignant neoplasms all sites	73
001–019	Tuberculosis	64
162–163	Malignant neoplasm of lung and bronchus	48
500–502	Bronchitis	23
	All causes	89

of the liver and suicide, and a much lower than average mortality from cancer (particularly lung cancer), bronchitis and tuberculosis. Their death rates from coronary disease and cerebrovascular disease are only a little higher than the national average.

STANDARD OF LIVING AND DISEASE

For more than a century it had been clear that standard of living has an important influence upon the pattern of mortality and morbidity, but the magnitude of the influence is difficult to measure. The concept of standard of living is complex and imprecise, including as it does housing, nutrition, education, recreation and many other inter-related influences. Family income would provide a good index of material prosperity but many difficulties stand in the way of collecting reliable information about it. A rough and ready measure of standard of living is provided by the occupation of the head of a family, as used by the Registrar General since the census of 1921. All occupations are divided into five 'social classes' on the basis of their standing in the community, the skill they demand and the income they command.

Class I   Higher professional and administrative occupations,
Class II Employers in industry and retail trades and the lesser professions,
Class III Skilled occupations,
Class IV Partly skilled occupations,
Class V   Unskilled occupations.

The classification is arbitrary and takes no account of personal circumstances (housing, family size, private income, etc.) other than those indicated by the stated occupation. Nevertheless it has provided much valuable information about the association between disease and social circumstances and is still a useful research tool.

Infant mortality increases regularly and sharply with social class, so that a child born into the family of an unskilled worker in 1961 was twice as likely to die in the first twelve months of life as a child born into a professional family. The same difference existed in 1921, but infant mortality has declined so much in all classes that in 1961 the infant in social class V had a better expectation of reaching its first birthday than the infant in social class I of forty years earlier.

That the percentage difference between mortality in class I and V should have remained about the same throughout a period when infant mortality as a whole declined dramatically was unexpected. In the first place welfare legislation (family allowances, food subsidies, national insurance, health services, local authority housing grants, etc.) has undoubtedly been of more benefit to the poorer sections of the community than to the well-to-do and this might have been expected to reduce the social gradient of infant mortality. And secondly, there was more scope for reduction of mortality from infection and other 'preventable' causes in class V than in class I. Yet because the percentage decline of total infant mortality has been about the same for both classes I and V, the proportionate decline from 'preventable' causes has evidently been greater for class I. Two possible influences may be mentioned in explanation of this apparent paradox: the better educated and well-to-do parents have earlier access to and make better use of social and medical advances; and there is more social mobility now than formerly, so that those in class V today are more likely to be there because of ill-health or lack of ability than those in class V forty years ago.

Some causes of first year death show much greater social class differentiation than infant mortality as a whole. The death rate from both gastroenteritis and pneumonia is five times greater in class V than in class I, a striking illustration of the importance of social circumstances in determining whether or not infants die from what are now treatable diseases.

In adult life the death rates for most of the major causes of death (including many of the malignancies) also increase from social class I to V. In a few exceptional and therefore particularly interesting cases the trend of the death rate in relation to social class is in the opposite direction, the professional classes having higher standardized mortality ratios than unskilled workers (table 20). Twenty years ago death rates from coronary disease were significantly higher in social class I and II than in IV and V. If anything the trend is now in the opposite direction; certainly it is for hypertension and vascular lesions of the C.N.S. The reverse trend for cholelithiasis and cholecystitis may be related to

Table 20. Standardized Mortality Ratios for certain causes by Social Class
(men aged 15–64, England and Wales 1959–63)

I.C.D. No.	Cause of Death	Social Class				
		I	II	III	IV	V
	(a) Examples of S.M.R.'s increasing with social class					
001–019	Tuberculosis	40	54	96	108	185
151	Malignant neoplasm of stomach	49	63	101	114	163
154	Malignant neoplasm of rectum	79	89	106	98	120
161	Malignant neoplasm of larynx	47	74	99	100	176
162, 163	Malignant neoplasm of lung, bronchus and trachea	53	72	107	104	148
330–334	Vascular lesions of CNS	86	89	101	98	135
410–416	Chronic rheumatic heart disease	67	69	104	110	146
420	Coronary disease, angina	98	95	106	96	112
440–447	Hypertension	85	96	99	96	138
490–493	Pneumonia	48	54	88	102	196
500–502	Bronchitis	28	50	97	116	194
541	Ulcer of duodenum	48	75	96	107	173
	(b) Examples of S.M.R.'s decreasing with social class					
178	Malignant neoplasm of testes	138	106	101	93	100
190	Melanoma of skin	150	116	100	95	84
451	Aortic aneurysm, non-syphilitic	132	110	105	91	89
584, 585	Cholelithiasis and cholecystitis	123	96	108	89	93

diet, but there is no obvious reason why the S.M.R. should be higher in the professional occupations than in the partly skilled and unskilled occupations for malignant disease of the testes, melanoma of the skin and non-syphilitic aortic aneurysm.

SEX DIFFERENCES IN DISEASE INCIDENCE

All countries with reasonably complete registration report an excess of males at birth (about 105 male for every 100 female infants). Throughout postnatal life, however, most death rates are higher for males than for females, with the result that in elderly populations there are normally more females than males. A measure of the sex difference in mortality is provided by expectation of life at birth, which in 1970 was six years less for males than for females (68·8 and 75·1 years respectively). It may be good fiscal policy, but it is otherwise anomalous that women should become pensionable at 60, when they have an expectation of a further 19·8 years of life; while men must wait until 65, by which time their expectation of life has dwindled to 12·0 years.

The reasons for the excess male mortality in postnatal life are complex. Table 21 shows that in England and Wales at the present time the heaviest contributions to the excess are made by ischaemic heart disease, bronchitis, cancer of the lung and road accidents. For these major causes of death much of the difference between the sexes is attributable to the different environments in which men and women live and work and to differences in their social habits (tobacco, alcohol, diet, occupation, etc.). On the other hand some of the variation in mortality experience is clearly biological in origin. Cancer of the breast and genital organs is much commoner in females, as are endocrinological (and particularly thyroid) disorders. The somewhat greater female mortality from cerebrovascular disease is due to the difference in age distribution, for at corresponding ages mortality is a little higher for males than for females. However, for many sex differences, there is so far no obvious explanation.

Although there are more liveborn males than females, more males than females are stillborn (about 105 to 100) and there is some evidence of an excess of male abortions. This suggests that more males than females are conceived. This possibility can be reconciled with the chromosome mechanism of sex determination, which supposes the

Table 21. Sex differences in mortality rates (England and Wales 1970)

I.C.D. No.	Some conditions with relatively high male mortality	Death rate per million		M/F
		Males	Females	
	Malignant neoplasm of:			
162	Trachea, bronchus, lung	1,045	214	4·9
188	Bladder	113	45	2·5
140–149	Buccal cavity and pharynx	42	27	1·6
151	Stomach	305	218	1·4
154	Rectum and rectosigmoid junction	130	109	1·2
490–493	Bronchitis, emphysema, asthma	928	321	2·9
010–019	Tuberculosis	47	19	2·5
E810–819	Motor vehicle traffic accidents	195	82	2·4
531–533	Peptic ulcer	96	58	1·7
410–414	Ischaemic heart disease	3,392	2,324	1·5
E950–959	Suicide	95	66	1·4

I.C.D. No.	Some conditions with relatively high female mortality	Death rate per million		F/M
		Males	Females	
	Malignant neoplasm of:			
174	Breast	3	424	141·3
193	Thyroid	5	11	2·2
180–186	Genital organs	179	319	1·8
156	Gall bladder and bile ducts	17	28	1·6
240–246	Thyroid disease other than neoplasm	4	20	5·0
E880–887	Accidental falls	76	152	2·0
156	Gall bladder and bile ducts, other than neoplasm	17	28	1·6
250	Diabetes mellitus	72	118	1·6
393–398	Chronic rheumatic heart disease	117	178	1·5
430–438	Cerebrovascular disease	1,294	1,926	1·5

production of equal numbers of X and Y bearing spermatozoa, by assuming the presence of sex-linked, gamete-lethal genes or of environmental influences affecting unequally the mobility or fertilizing ability of the two types of spermatozoa. It is not certain, however, that there is an excess of males at conception. More males than females are stillborn; but among stillbirths three times more females than males have gross malformations of the central nervous system (anencephaly and spina bifida). Information about the sex-ratio of abortions, although suggesting an excess of males, is not very reliable, for collections of early embryos are almost always unrepresentative. In view of the high abortion rates in early pregnancy, no great excess of females among early abortions would be required to make the observed preponderance of males at birth consistent with equal numbers of males and females at conception.

Although mortality is higher for males than females throughout life, the reverse appears to be true of morbidity. Certainly general practititioner consultations, hospital admissions and sickness surveys all show a considerable excess of females. The reasons are even more complex than the reasons for the mortality differences. It does not follow that women are more often sick or disabled although some studies suggest that they are. The explanation may lie in part in a sex difference in awareness of minor departures from health, and in readiness to seek medical advice. And since fewer women are in full-time employment, they have more opportunity to consult their general practitioners.

FURTHER READING

Morris J. N. (1964) *The Uses of Epidemiology*, 2nd Edition. E. & S. Livingstone, Edinburgh.

6 · INTERNATIONAL VARIATION IN DISEASE INCIDENCE

For many parts of the world there is little information about morbidity and even mortality data are unreliable. The World Health Organization has done much to standardize methods of registering and recording deaths and the *International Statistical Classification of Diseases, Injuries and Causes of Death* has been generally adopted (Chapter 32). However, in many countries births and deaths are under-registered, stated cause of death is unreliable and population censuses are at irregular intervals and incomplete. Nevertheless, it is quite clear that there are differences in mortality between countries at least as large as between nineteenth and twentieth century Britain and a great deal larger than the regional or social class differences demonstrable today. For example, in 1970 infant mortality in Scandinavia was less than fifteen per 1,000 live births (in England and Wales it was eighteen); but in many countries it was over 50 (figure 9), and in parts of Africa, South America and South East Asia it was probably over 200.

A medical opinion on cause of death is necessary before any reliance can be placed on a country's analysis of its deaths, but unfortunately in those parts of the world where death rates are high, many deaths are not attended by a physician. (In England and Wales there is one qualified medical practitioner to 800 of the population, in India there is one to 6,000 and in parts of Africa one to 100,000.) Clearly international comparisons of cause of mortality have to be interpreted with caution.

However, certain differences are immediately obvious. In developed countries such as England and Wales, arteriosclerotic heart disease and malignancies are the leading causes of death and account together for more than half of all deaths. Infectious disease is relatively unimportant accounting for less than one per cent of deaths. In the developing countries of Africa, South East Asia and Latin America the pattern is reversed. Cancer and heart disease together account only for one death in ten, and infectious diseases make by far the biggest contribution to mortality, accounting for one third of all deaths.

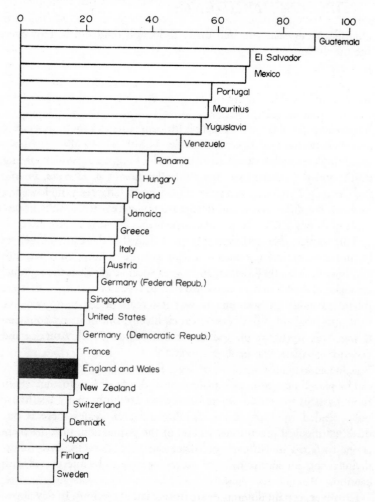

Figure 9. Infant mortality in selected countries, 1970.

CAUSES OF INTERNATIONAL DIFFERENCES

We have seen that climatic differences may explain part of the increase in mortality from the south east to the north west of the British Isles. Climate might therefore be expected to have some influence on the international pattern or mortality. Malaria remains one of the most important causes of death and disability in the world. Although the disease is being brought slowly under control, many millions have clinical attacks each year and many thousands die from it. However, the anopheline mosquitoes which transmit the disease require particular geographical and climatic conditions for breeding, and minimum temperature needs have to be met before the plasmodium can complete its life cycle within the mosquito. Consequently the influence of the disease upon world mortality is limited by climate and geography. There is no malaria in the Arctic circle or the Sahara.

Yellow fever and trypanosomiasis also kill and disable on a large scale. They are even more closely confined by geography and climate than malaria. Yellow fever depends for its life cycle on an ecology of animal host, insect vector, temperature, humidity and plant life peculiar to the tropical rain forests of Africa and Central and South America, and trypanosomiasis is confined to the bush of Africa.

The spread of many other infectious diseases, although not geographically limited, is favoured by particular climatic conditions. For example, in hot climates flies contribute to the spread of bowel infections, while in cold climates crowding at home, school, work and places of entertainment encourages the dissemination of air-borne infection. The climatic influence is not restricted to infectious disease: rickets was formerly predominantly a disease of countries that are short of sunshine, and chronic bronchitis is above all a disease of coal burning industrialization.

Clearly climate and geography play a part in determining international differences in experience of disease, disability and death. Much more important, however, is the stage of economic and social development. Within limits, mortality from infectious disease can be lowered to the extent that a government is able and willing to pay for the appropriate public health and medical services. Leprosy, plague, smallpox, typhus and cholera, now thought of as tropical diseases, were all at one time common in Britain. Tuberculosis is fast disappearing from Europe and North America and will soon become a 'tropical' disease. In the eighteenth and nineteenth centuries malaria and yellow fever made West Africa the white man's grave. It has been suggested that if northern Europe had been colonized from Africa, rickets and respiratory infections would have made Britain the black man's grave.

Two examples can be given of the relative insignficance of climate in determining the level of mortality. In South Africa infant mortality in 1961 was 27 for the white population, 42 for the Asiatic (largely Indian) population and 125 for the 'Coloured' population. The rate for the native Bantu was not known, but it was certainly higher than the rate for coloured infants.

It has often been suggested that there are racial differences in susceptibility to disease due to differences in genetic constitution. Tuberculosis is usually cited as an example, but even for this disease the evidence is inconclusive. White, Indian and coloured infants in South Africa are subject to the same climatic conditions, and the differences in their mortality experience may be in part genetically determined. But the contribution of genes is negligible compared to that of nutrition, standard of housing, sanitation, water supply and medical and welfare services.

The second example is provided by comparison of mortality from cardiovascular and malignant disease in Scotland and Sweden, two countries lying at similar latitudes and with populations of much the same size. In 1961 for both groups of diseases the death rate among men aged 55–64 in Sweden was half that in Scotland and for cancer of the lung the Swedish death rate was only one-fifth of the Scottish rate. Climate and genetics can have little to do with these differences and they must be due largely to social, economic and industrial factors. For example the populations of the two countries differ substantially in their smoking, drinking, eating and exercise habits; and Sweden with no large industrialized areas, and little use of coal, has smaller and cleaner towns and cities than Scotland.

PRESENT POSITION AND FUTURE TRENDS

At the present time different countries are at very different stages of the so-called demographic cycle. They can be grouped into four broad categories according to their mortality and natality experience.
(a) Countries in which both birth rate and death rate are still high and

malnutrition and infectious disease remain the leading causes of death (parts of Africa, South East Asia and Latin America).
(b) Countries in which the birth rate is still high but the death rate is now falling (India and parts of Latin America).
(c) Countries in which the birth rate is declining and the death rate is falling very rapidly (Ceylon, Taiwan and Mauritius).
(d) Countries in which both birth rate and death rate are low, cardiovascular and malignant disease are the leading causes of death and infection is no longer important (the countries of Northern Europe, North America and Japan).

With the exception of Japan, as the countries in the last category passed through the preceding phases of the demographic cycle, their progression from high to low mortality occurred over two centuries. Many countries of the world are now crowding this experience into two generations. In Britain the fall in mortality was well under way before public environmental and personal health services were introduced and long before the advent of effective specific prevention and treatment of the major infections. The accumulated knowledge and experience of the western world is being applied to less developed countries with dramatic results. For example, the crude mortality rate in Japan immediately before the war was 17·4 per thousand (the level of mortality in England and Wales in the last decade of the nineteenth century); by 1970 it had fallen to 6·9 (in the same year the mortality of our much older population was 11·7).

Increase in world population

The population of the world doubled from about 500 million in 1630 to 1,000 million in 1830. It doubled again over the next one hundred years to reach about 2,000 million in 1930; by 1975 it will have doubled once more to reach 4,000 million, and if the present rate of growth continues (slightly over two per cent per year) it will double yet again to reach 8,000 million by about the year 2010.

Another consequence of high birth rates and falling death rates is a change in the age structure. One of the most striking differences between developed and developing countries is in the proportion of children in the population. For example in Europe about 20 per cent of the population are under fifteen compared with 45 per cent in Africa and Latin America.

In 1789 Malthus published his *Essay on the Principle of Population*.

His main thesis was that food production can never keep pace with natural fertility so that population growth is inevitably checked by famine and epidemic disease: 'The power of the population is so superior to the power in the earth to produce subsistence for man, that premature death must in some shape or other visit the human race. The vices of mankind are active and able ministers of depopulation. They are the precursors in the great army of destruction and often finish the dreadful work themselves. But should they fail in this war of extermination, sickly seasons, epidemics, pestilence and plague advance in terrific array. Should success be incomplete, gigantic inevitable famine stalks in the rear, and with one mighty blow levels the population with the food of the world.'

Since Malthus's time there has been a fivefold increase in the population of England and Wales and standard of living has much more than kept pace with the increase. The disasters he predicted have not occurred because our lead in production of machine-made goods made it possible to buy enough food from abroad to meet the needs of an expanding population. But the Malthusian principle remains valid. There is no reliable information about the proportion of people now existing on a diet below minimum physiological needs, but it is probably not less (and may be considerably more) than one-quarter of the world's population. In India about twentyfive millions died of famine in the last quarter of the nineteenth century (the equivalent of the total population of England and Wales at that time), and five millions died in the disastrous Bengal famine in 1945.

From rough estimates it would seem that during the twentieth century world food supplies have barely kept pace with the growth of population. Food production is still increasing and is likely to increase even more. The total area under cultivation has been extended; improved strains of seed and cattle developed and better systems of cultivation, with mechanization and more effective use of fertilizers introduced; waste from soil erosion, animal pests and microorganisms reduced; freshwater and saltwater fish bred for food; and there is much experiment in the field of biochemical engineering to produce food, and especially proteins, by laboratory methods. But all this will be ineffective unless birth rates are lowered. Western experience suggests that improved living conditions eventually lead to a voluntary decrease in a nation's birth rate, but this is a slow process and it is questionable whether food production can be increased rapidly enough to feed the expanding world population until this happens.

FURTHER READING

BROCKINGTON C. F. (1967) *World Health*, 2nd Edition. J. & A. Churchill Ltd, London.

PART II

Means

CONTROL OF INHERITANCE

7 · CONTROL OF THE GENETIC CONSTITUTION OF HUMAN POPULATIONS

CONTROL OF BREEDING

When they wish to improve their stocks, plant and animal breeders do not hesitate to manipulate the environment, or to control reproduction by selection of one or both parents. Choice between these methods is determined by effectiveness and cost. The marked improvement in the quality of livestock which followed the introduction of root crops in the eighteenth century is an example of the first method; the modern thoroughbred racehorse and improvements in the protein content of maize are examples of the second.

It should be noted that the use of selection as a means of improving crops and livestock preceded the establishment of the science of genetics. To farmers who knew nothing of genes and chromosomes it was clearly worthwhile to select parents on the basis of their characteristics or those of their offspring. In practice this procedure has not been greatly altered by genetical knowledge. Breeders of racehorses still assess the value of a sire according to both his record in competition and the performance of his offspring.

The characteristics of human beings have also been determined by selection. Infectious disease, for example, must have had a profound influence on human evolution, since it killed large numbers of people—until recently the majority of those born—before they could reproduce. There is, however, an important difference between this kind of selection and the purposeful selection practised by farmers. There has been no conscious control of human reproduction, and to a visitor from

Mars it would no doubt seem remarkable that men have not applied to their own kind the methods which have had such conspicuous success with plants and other animals. We shall consider the reasons for this restraint in relation to three themes: ethics; effectiveness; and desirability.

Ethics

The first question is an ethical one: Would it be right to control human breeding? It is not surprising that there are wide differences of opinion about the answer. On religious grounds some people believe that in no circumstances would it be right to interfere with the 'natural' pattern of reproduction. Others consider that the evolution of the human race is too important to be determined by the sexual attraction between two individuals, and that human beings should eventually transfer their reproductive functions to the laboratory.

These are extreme views and most people take an intermediate position. While they do not object in principle to some control of breeding, they are concerned about the methods of achieving it and the purposes for which it is to be employed. They are particularly doubtful about the use of compulsory powers.

Effectiveness

The second question to be considered is whether control of breeding would be effective. This question must be made more precise. Would it be possible either to eliminate or reduce the frequency of undesirable genotypes, or to increase the frequency of desirable genotypes? In relation to the first question we shall refer separately to the few conditions which appear to be attributable to a single gene, and to the much larger number, including most important diseases, which are not.

With due regard for a reservation (mutation) referred to below, in the case of conditions due to a single gene the effectiveness of suppressing reproduction depends upon the extent to which it is possible to identify those who carry the gene. By preventing reproduction of affected persons it would be possible to eliminate dominant genotypes which are completely manifested before reproductive age. This requirement is more or less met in only a few rare abnormalities, for example in achondroplasia, and in a certain type of juvenile cataract. In most dominant genotypes the requirement is not met, either because the abnormality is not completely manifested in all environments, or because it does not appear until after reproduction. Huntington's chorea is an example of a condition due to a dominant gene which cannot be eliminated in this manner because it becomes evident in middle life when those affected may have reproduced.

As a rule single genes which cause abnormalities are recessive, and manifested only in the homozygous state. The number of individuals who carry the gene but are not themselves affected (the heterozygotes) is much larger than the number of affected (the homozygotes). For example only about 1 in 20,000 individuals exhibit albinism (i.e. are homozygous), whereas about 1 in 70 carry the gene but are not affected (are heterozygous). Hence only a small proportion of those affected have affected parents, the suppression of whose reproduction would have relatively little effect on the frequency of the gene. Reduction of the incidence of a sex-linked recessive condition, such as haemophilia, would be more feasible, but would require restriction of breeding of daughters and sisters of affected males, as well as of the affected males themselves.

We have so far ignored the fact that genetically-determined abnormalities also result from mutation, the reservation referred to above. The mutation rates so far estimated in man are relatively low, but they are by no means insignificant. In haemophilia, for example, the frequency of mutation is apparently high enough to maintain the incidence of the disease at a fairly constant level, in spite of the fact that until recently most affected males died before reproductive age. Control of reproduction would not reduce the incidence of a genetic condition below the level which results from mutation.

In most human diseases the genetic mechanisms are not established. But it is clear that they are not attributable to a single gene, and that they are influenced to a considerable degree by the environment. There is therefore no basis for exact prediction of the effects of control of reproduction although in most cases they would undoubtedly be small. For example, most mentally subnormal persons have normal parents, and prevention of reproduction of those affected would have little influence on the incidence of mental subnormality in the general population.

It is even less certain that control of breeding would make it possible to increase the frequency of desirable genotypes. There are some qualities—honesty, intelligence, vitality, etc.—which most people would regard as desirable. But little is known about the respective contributions of inheritance and environment in determining these qualities, and nothing is known about the related genes. It seems probable that if parents were selected with no other object than an increase in stature it could soon be achieved. It is far from certain that the same is true of intelligence, or of the other unmeasured, and perhaps unmeasurable, qualities regarded as desirable. Moreover although cattle are bred with a single object such as increased milk yield or improved quality of beef, no single object would be acceptable in man. It is also conceivable that improvement of one feature might be accompanied by deterioration of another.

We may summarize our conclusions about the possibility of control of human inheritance by quoting a statement by a group of well-known geneticists. 'At the present level of genetic knowledge we cannot improve the genes with which we are born, and there is little we can do to determine which genes we pass on to our children.'

Desirability

Finally, if it were permissible and effective, would it be desirable to control human inheritance? Again the question must be put more precisely. No one is likely to quarrel with the statement that the elimination of many genetically-determined diseases and abnormalities would be desirable if brought about by acceptable methods. But some people also suggest that it would be useful to increase the proportion of genetically well-endowed people. This claim requires closer scrutiny.

The belief that it would be desirable to increase the proportion of gifted people presupposes that improvement in human affairs is at present restricted by lack of them. It is difficult to accept this view. The fact that achievement has been outstanding only in certain places and for short periods—in Italy during the Renaissance, for example—suggests that at most times the environment is unfavourable. (The alternative explanation—that there have been some remarkable mutations at different times in history—is not credible.) Hence it seems probable that there is a large reserve of ability which is not exploited.

Moreover it might not be possible to provide suitable employment and rewards for a larger number of gifted people. There are perhaps few jobs which could not be done better by intelligent than by less intelligent people; but many occupations already demand abilities which they do not fully reward and others give little satisfaction because they do not use fully the capacities of those employed in them. Modification of the proportion of individuals with different levels of ability might therefore create more problems than it would solve.

EUGENIC PRACTICE

Francis Galton (1822–1911) introduced the word eugenics in reference to 'the study of agencies under social control, that may improve or impair the racial (i.e. inherited) qualities of future generations, either physically or mentally'. Galton's views about how this was to be done changed considerably during his own lifetime, as he became more aware of difficulties. In general his emphasis passed from the negative to the positive aspect of the subject; from concern about those who should not breed, to interest in those who should. This trend has characterized the eugenics movement, which is now particularly interested in social policies which might encourage desirable parents to have larger families.

The discussion which follows is concerned with the limitation of genetic disease. We shall consider three approaches, prevention of conception, abortion, and withholding treatment of affected individuals after birth—measures which may be summarized pithily if not quite accurately as gametocide, feticide, and infanticide. It should be noted that in the progression from conception to pregnancy to birth, the ethical acceptability of intervention diminishes (contraception is more acceptable than abortion and abortion than infanticide). But in the same progression the effectiveness of the procedures increases, for whereas infanticide can be restricted to abnormal births, limitation of genetic disease by feticide, and still more by gametocide, prevents the birth of a considerable number of normal individuals. Since the relative specificities of the three procedures are known, the choice between them is more an ethical than a technical matter.

Prevention of conception

(a) *Compulsory.* The most severe measure is sterilization of persons believed to be unfit to reproduce. It is not practised in Britain, but has been used in Germany, and in the United States a majority of the States have laws which permit or require sterilization of individuals affected by certain conditions. About twentyfour conditions are included, but as each American State makes its own decision, only a few are common to most States—idiocy, imbecility, feeblemindedness, insanity, and epilepsy. We should note three points about these classes. In the first place, none of them is a genetic entity; for example, the mentally subnormal include a few types which have a simple genetic basis, and a very much larger number which do not. Secondly, with perhaps the exception of epilepsy, little or nothing is known about the genetic background of the majority of cases included in each class. And thirdly, it is very doubtful whether suppression of reproduction of affected persons would have much effect on the incidence of the defects. It should of course be said that sterilization is sometimes advocated not only on genetic grounds, but also on the social grounds that individuals suffering from these conditions are incapable of providing a reasonable home environment for their children.

An alternative method used to suppress reproduction is to segregate affected individuals, at least during their reproductive years. This procedure makes it possible to provide supervision and care; but since it requires separation of the sexes, and restriction of leave, it is an open question whether it is more humane than sterilization. If a choice is to be made between segregation and sterilization, it seems most reasonable to base it upon the affected individual's need for institutional care rather than upon the relative effectiveness of the two methods in suppressing reproduction.

(b) *Voluntary.* Another approach to eugenic practice is the provision of advice to parents or prospective parents about the risk of occurrence of undesirable traits in their children. The question may be raised by persons about to be married, by married couples contemplating pregnancy, or by a woman who is pregnant. The common reasons for concern are that parents or prospective parents are closely related (usually they are cousins); that one or both have an undesirable trait; or that previous children or other relatives have had such a trait.

The restriction of disease by discouraging parents likely to have affected offspring seemed a realistic policy when genes were believed to be numbered in thousands rather than millions, and when a clear distinction between normal and abnormal genes was thought to be possible. Recent knowledge of the nature of genetic disease has made it difficult to see how a population can benefit substantially from attempts to influence fertility on medical grounds. This approach is feasible in the rare disorders due to dominant genes; it may also have a limited use after the birth of an abnormality such as anencephalus, whose genetical background is obscure, but for which increased risk of recurrence in later children of the same sibship has been estimated empirically. But even if applied consistently such restrictions on reproduction could make only a trivial contribution to the prevention of disease; moreover, as noted above they would lead to the prevention of a large number of normal pregnancies.

Abortion

Although fetal diagnosis has long been practised by obstetricians concerned with the management of pregnancy and labour, it has only recently been extended to identification of genetic disorders by amniocentesis. But from the time (1956) when it became possible to define the sex of the fetus from the presence or absence of sex chromatin in fetal cells in the amniotic fluid, it was recognized that methods might be developed which would permit the identification and abortion of some abnormal embryos. Since then fetal cells have been shown to be capable of multiplication in vitro, allowing the study of any characteristics revealed by tissue culture, either in the cytoplasm or the nuclei, in addition to the analysis of the amniotic fluid. These methods can now be used in chromosomal disorders, such as mongolism and in certain genic disorders, such as Tay-Sachs disease and gargoylism. At present, they are impractical in the commoner conditions such as fibrocystic disease, phenylketonuria and haemoglobinopathies.

Unfortunately there are considerable difficulties in making full use of this knowledge. In the first place, the procedure is practicable only from the 14th week of pregnancy, when amniocentesis becomes reasonably safe, until the 16th week, when abortion becomes difficult. And secondly, screening of all pregnancies is not at present feasible, and when investigation is restricted to pregnancies of mothers who have had an abnormal birth, the reduction in the frequency of chromosomal and genic disorders is relatively small. Indeed some of those who have had extensive experience of amniocentesis consider that its limited benefits do not justify inclusion of the technique and subsequent abortion as part of normal clinical practice. Its value is undoubtedly greatest in relation to a condition such as haemophilia, where a substantial reduction in incidence could be achieved by preventing haemophiliacs having daughters.

Withholding treatment after birth

The procedures referred to above have four major limitations: (a) even if fully applied they would not prevent the conception and birth of a large number of abnormal children; (b) their full application would require avoidance of conception or abortion of many normal individuals; (c) amniocentesis followed by abortion involves risks for the mother which, if not great, are not negligible; and (d) amniocentesis without abortion may expose the fetus to some risk.

These objections are absent or much less serious in the case of infanticide. This procedure does not require destruction of normal births and presents no physical risks to the mother. It is true that not all major abnormalities can be recognized soon after birth, but the proportion missed is much smaller than before or during pregnancy. The objections to infanticide as a means of eliminating serious malformations are essentially of a personal and ethical kind. The loss of a child after birth is much more stressful for parents than contraception or abortion. And death of live births is unacceptable on ethical grounds, particularly when it is caused by active measures, but also to some people when it results from withholding treatment. These issues were discussed in Chapter 2.

FURTHER READING

Bresler J. B. (ed.) (1973) *Genetics and Society*. Addison Wesley Publishing Co., Reading, Mass.

Burnet M. (1971) *Genes, Dreams and Realities*. Medical and Technical Publishing Co., Ltd., Aylesbury, Bucks.

Dobzhansky T. (1946) *Heredity and the Nature of Man*. Harcourt, Brace and World, New York.

PERSONAL MEASURES

8 · IMMUNIZATION

In medical teaching there has been some uncertainty about responsibility for instruction in immunization and we must begin by clarifying our interpretation of it. Discussion of the organisms which cause infectious disease is clearly the concern of departments of bacteriology and virology. Clinical departments should deal with the clinical manifestations of the infections and, we suggest, with the immunization procedures used to prevent them. Formerly these subjects were often discussed by teachers of preventive medicine and public health, and this was perhaps justified when they were specialists in infectious disease. These circumstances have changed. Many teachers of social medicine have had little clinical experience of infection and it seems best to regard the prevention of infectious disease in the individual, like its treatment, as the concern of clinical medicine.

Our task in social medicine is to evaluate the contribution of immunization. It has long been recognized that those who recover from infectious illness frequently acquire some degree of protection, and the Chinese attempted to exploit this knowledge by inoculating with material from mild cases of smallpox. This hazardous procedure was introduced to the British Isles in 1721 and appears to have been employed fairly extensively in the eighteenth century. It was replaced by cowpox vaccination from 1798, the first example of safe and effective immunization and the only one for nearly a hundred years. The identification of bacteria led to the use of antitoxin for treatment of diphtheria from 1891. With these exceptions immunization procedures were developed in the present century, and used widely in Britain only after 1940.

For the purpose of evaluating the contribution of immunization we shall first consider diseases against which immunization is now routinely employed in Britain, and secondly diseases in which vaccines are not offered routinely but are administered in certain circumstances.

ROUTINE IMMUNIZATION

Diphtheria

Mortality from diphtheria in England and Wales has declined fairly continuously since the late nineteenth century (figure 10). It was then a relatively common cause of death in children. Today it is a rare disease, and many doctors who have qualified since the end of the Second World War have never seen it. In the six years, 1965–70, there were only nine deaths from diphtheria in England and Wales.

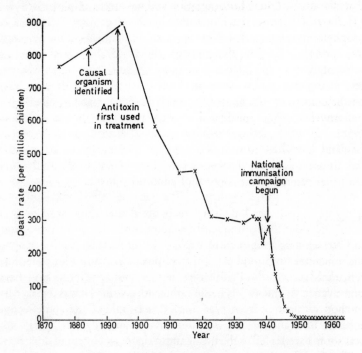

Figure 10. Diphtheria. Mean annual death rate of children under 15: England and Wales.

It is not possible to assess with any precision the relative importance of the various influences which have contributed to the decline of mortality from the disease. Antitoxin was first used in the late nineteenth century and has been the accepted form of treatment since that time. It is believed to have reduced the case fatality rate, which fell from 8·2 per 100 notifications in 1916–25 to 5·4 in 1933–42, while notifications remained at an average level of above 50,000 per year in England and Wales. The mortality rate increased at the beginning of the last war, but fell rapidly at about the time when national immunization was introduced (figure 10).

It is tempting to attribute much of the decline of diphtheria mortality between 1895 and 1922 to treatment by antitoxin, and the rapid fall since 1940 to immunization. Nothing in the evidence is seriously inconsistent with this interpretation, and if mortality from the other common infections had increased or even remained constant in the same period it could possibly be accepted unreservedly. But the fact that diseases such as whooping cough (figure 11) and measles (figure 13) showed a large reduction of mortality, without treatment or prophylaxis, suggests that other unspecified influences were at work. We cannot exclude the possibility that they also contributed, perhaps substantially, to the decline of diphtheria. With due regard for this reservation it seems probable that immunization has had more effect on the control of this disease than of any other, with the exception of poliomyelitis. This conclusion is supported by the high level of immunity which follows the use of a good antigen. Evidence for England and Wales in 1961–63 suggested that the risk of an attack of the disease was about six times greater, and the risk of a fatal attack ten times greater, in those not immunized than in the immunized.

Tuberculosis

In Chapter 1 we discussed the trend of mortality from tuberculosis in the nineteenth century (figure 4) and the possible reasons for its remarkable decline. Attempts to protect by vaccination began in 1890, when Koch introduced tuberculin, an extract of dead bacteria. The method was unsuccessful, and was followed by use of living virulent tubercle bacilli. This procedure was recognized to be dangerous and was soon abandoned.

The first avirulent live vaccine, and the one in general use today was B.C.G. (Bacille Calmette-Guérin). The bovine strain was virulent when first isolated (in 1906), but rapidly lost its virulence when cultured on potato with added ox bile. Although Calmette and Guérin first described the strain in 1908, it was not administered as a prophylactic in man until 1921, or generally released before 1924. For a few years it was used mainly in France and Scandinavia, where it was given almost exclusively to children of tuberculous parents and to tuberculin-negative adults considered to be exposed to special risks of acquiring the disease.

The policy of vaccinating tuberculin-negative individuals in the general population was accepted in Scandinavia in about 1940 and has since spread to many other countries. In Britain B.C.G. was used from 1949 for persons exposed to special risks of tuberculosis, and in 1953 the Ministry of Health recommended vaccination of all tuberculin-negative children at age 13. By this time mortality from respiratory tuberculosis in England and Wales had declined to less than one-fifteenth of its level when first registered (figure 4).

The value of B.C.G. vaccination has been assessed recently by Springett, and the following discussion is based largely on his conclusions.

If all members of a community are tuberculin positive, or if all are tuberculin negative, B.C.G. vaccination is useless: in the first case because all are already infected; in the second because none can become infected. Between these theoretical extreme possibilities the value of B.C.G. must be assessed in relation to the extent to which it reduces the incidence of tuberculosis in vaccinated negatives as compared with those left unvaccinated. In a number of trials tuberculosis morbidity or mortality was between 30 per cent and 80 per cent lower in those vaccinated than in controls. The large difference between the results was probably due to variation in the circumstances of each trial. The type of vaccine and the conditions under which it is used are therefore important.

Low levels of protection do not justify a vaccination campaign, and a 75 per cent reduction of morbidity or mortality should be the objective. Conclusions concerning the use of B.C.G. in circumstances which are common in the world today are as follows.

1. *Many tuberculin positives and high conversion rate.* Conditions still to be found in many countries of the world, especially where facilities for treatment are limited. It seems certain that B.C.G. vaccination can effectively reduce the amount of tuberculosis under these conditions,

and the main problem is to decide to which groups to offer it. In most communities of this type, very large numbers of adolescents are tuberculin positive, and the only logical use for B.C.G. is its application to all new-born children, as at no other age is the uninfected population large enough for B.C.G. to be fully effective.

2. *Percentage positive high, but infection rate falling from previously very high levels.* The situation of many countries with well developed tuberculosis services with full utilization of adequate chemotherapy. The factor of greatest importance here is the conversion rate to be expected in negatives; if the great majority of children are reaching adolescence tuberculin negative, then the most effective use for B.C.G. on a community scale would be at about the age of puberty, to protect against the increase of tuberculosis experienced in adolescence and young adult life. As infection rates fall still further, the final stage may be reached of:

3. *Percentage positive low.* With declining infection rates a point is reached when the disadvantages of artificial tuberculin conversion and the cost of the procedure no longer justify its use. It is probable that some parts of the world with well developed health services and good living conditions have already reached this stage.

These three types of circumstances are to be found in under-developed countries (1), in technologically advanced countries (or in sub-groups of the population within them) where infection rates are not low (2), and in technologically advanced countries where infection rates are low (3).

The issues are complex in the first type of community, where infection is common, medical resources are limited, and social and economic conditions are poor. In such circumstances the grounds for prevention of disease are even stronger than in developed countries (because treatment is less likely to be available), but the widespread use of vaccination raises three questions.

1. How effective is B.C.G. in undeveloped societies? In countries such as Britain, vaccination was not used until mortality had declined to a small fraction of its initial level (figure 4), by which time the population had a relatively high standard of living and malnutrition was very uncommon. However, experience in Algeria, Southern India and North America (with Indian populations) suggests that even in very different conditions B.C.G. remains relatively effective.

2. Would the use of B.C.G. prejudice the application of other methods, particularly improved housing and diet? These measures are very effective, and it would be a serious loss if the use of specific protection resulted in their neglect.

3. Does vaccination make the best use of a limited number of medical and other trained workers? In a country where tuberculosis is common B.C.G. is undoubtedly to be preferred to treatment, particularly since it needs only a single procedure, carried out by a team which may not include a doctor. The question is more difficult where the ratio of trained workers to population is very low, as it still is in many countries. There the most urgent tasks for the doctor and his associates are probably to teach, to plan and to administer; and a specific procedure which leads to the neglect of these services is bought dearly.

The value of B.C.G. in the second and third types of community referred to above can be assessed fairly accurately, the main problem being to decide at what point vaccination is no longer justified. Certainly it should be continued so long as the cost of treating and maintaining cases which could be prevented is greater than the cost of giving B.C.G. to the whole population (or group). But when the cost of vaccination exceeds the cost of case-finding, treatment and maintenance, the question becomes more difficult, not least because the answer cannot be decided solely on economic grounds.

It has been estimated that in Britain in 1969–70 the percentage of children infected at age 13 was 8 per cent, and at this level it was considered desirable to immunize routinely children aged 10–13. However the percentage infected is still falling, and it will soon reach a level where B.C.G. will be contributing little to the control of tuberculosis. Long before the end of the century it will probably be decided that vaccination should no longer be used routinely. It will still be desirable to have selective programmes for groups exposed to special risks, such as hospital workers and possibly people going abroad to areas where there is an appreciable risk of tuberculous infection.

Whooping cough

Figure 11 shows the trend of mortality from whooping cough expressed as the annual death rate of children under 15. In the mid-nineteenth century this disease was a very frequent cause of death, particularly in young children; about as frequent as measles and very much more so than poliomyelitis in the present century. Mortality has declined almost continuously since about 1870, and there are now few deaths in England and Wales (fifteen in 1970 of which thirteen were in children under 1 year).

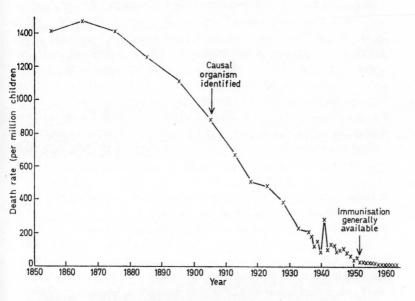

Figure 11. Whooping cough. Mean annual death rate of children under 15: England and Wales.

The causal organism, *Bordetella pertussis*, was identified in 1906. Immunization is complicated by the fact that the organism has multiple serotypes, and a child may be infected simultaneously with two or more of them. Moreover the potency of vaccines is not constant, and the protective effect of vaccination has been observed to vary between less than 30 per cent and over 80 per cent. Current practice is to immunize children routinely from the age of three months.

No convincing explanation can be given for the great reduction of mortality from whooping cough since the mid-nineteenth century. Treatment by sulphonamides and (later) antibiotics was not available before 1939, and even now its effect on the course of the disease is questionable. Immunization can have contributed little, for it was not available until 1952, by which time mortality in England and Wales had declined to a small fraction of its level in 1872.

Poliomyelitis

Poliomyelitis appears to have been a rare disease before the late nineteenth century, but since that time it has occurred in epidemics in many countries. It is due to a virus which infects the alimentary tract and only occasionally causes the paralysis which is a striking feature of the disease; it is important to recognize that the number of cases infected but with few or no clinical manifestations exceeds greatly (by about 100 to 1) the number of cases affected by paralysis. In its paralytic form poliomyelitis presents the anomaly of an intestinal infection whose incidence increases as social conditions improve, for it is most common in countries with a high standard of living. An explanation which can be offered with reservations is that in primitive conditions children acquire immunity by early exposure to the infection (the polio virus is endemic in communities which lack hygiene), whereas if hygiene is good they are protected from exposure and hence less resistant when they meet the disease in adult life. It is consistent with this interpretation that although the disease is most common in young children, its clinical manifestations are most severe in adults.

Because of the conspicuous disabilities which are common in patients who survive, there is, understandably, some tendency to overestimate the significance of poliomyelitis in relation to other infections. In 1947, when the highest death rate was recorded in England and Wales, there were 33 deaths from the disease per million children under 15 (figure 12) compared with 99 from whooping cough and 69 from measles. In 1871–80, before the decline of mortality began, the last two diseases were responsible for 1,415 and 1,038 deaths (per million under 15) respectively.

Poliomyelitis was recognized as an infection in 1909 and shown to be due to a filterable virus. Two methods of immunization have been used widely: inactivated vaccine containing killed virus (Salk); and live attenuated virus vaccine (Sabin). The former was in use in Britain from 1956, but the latter is generally preferred since it can be given orally and the immunity conferred is greater and lasts longer. Moreover the attenuated viruses of the oral vaccine result in antibody formation in the blood and local resistance to subsequent infection with virulent poliomyelitis viruses. This reduces the number of symptomless excreters of virulent poliomyelitis virus in the community.

Figure 12 shows the time (1956) when immunization against poliomyelitis became common in England and Wales. On this evidence alone, particularly because of the variation in mortality before 1956, it would be impossible to assess the contribution of immunization. Nevertheless there are grounds for believing that it is very effective. Laboratory evidence indicates that it gives a high degree of immunity, as measured by the titre of circulating antibody. Results of controlled trials have been impressive. And poliomyelitis has been almost eliminated from countries which have had effective immunization programmes, whereas it is still common in countries which have not. A surveillance scheme in existence in England and Wales shows that a slight risk of poliomyelitis induced by the oral vaccine cannot be ruled out, but the risk is considered to be so small that it does not justify restriction on the vaccination programme.

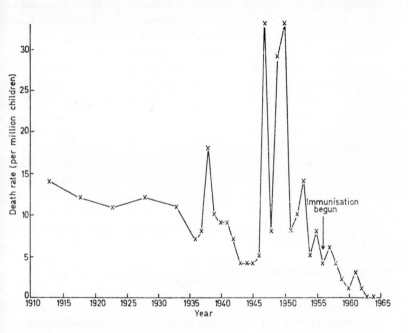

Figure 12. Poliomyelitis. Mean annual death rate of children under 15: England and Wales.

Measles

During the nineteenth and early twentieth centuries childhood mortality from measles was relatively high, but it declined rapidly from about the time of the First World War (figure 13). Nevertheless measles remains an important infectious disease; in 1970 nearly 300,000 cases were notified in England and there were 40 deaths.

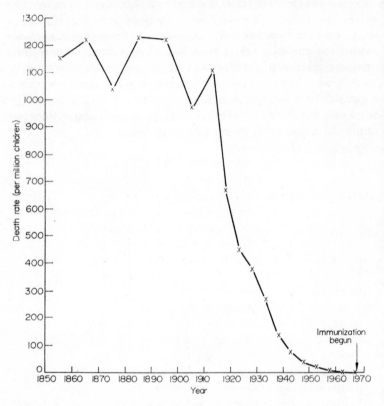

Figure 13. Measles. Mean annual death rate of children under 15: England and Wales.

It is now recommended that children should be immunized routinely with a vaccine containing live attenuated measles virus. In trials the living vaccine produced antibody in 95 per cent of those vaccinated and a Medical Research Council protection trial suggested that the procedure was over 90 per cent effective. On this and other evidence it was hoped that it might be possible to eradicate measles, and it was estimated that vaccination of 75 per cent or more of children at one year of age would result in control of the disease. The success expected has not yet been achieved, partly perhaps because the requirements for it have not been met fully. In both the United Kingdom and the United States extensive vaccination programmes have changed the epidemic pattern of measles and appear to have lowered its incidence but they have not prevented the reappearance of epidemics. Among the reasons suggested for this disappointing result are failure to vaccinate enough children, unsatisfactory vaccination (due for example to the lability of the vaccine or to the fact that it is administered too early in life), and waning of immunity which is observed with certain strains. Nevertheless some epidemiologists remain convinced that eradication of measles could be achieved if the proportion of children immunized were high enough.

Whatever doubts there may be about the contribution of vaccination to the control of measles during the last four years it is clear that it cannot have contributed to the decline of incidence or mortality in Britain before 1968 when it was first used widely. No convincing explanation has been given for the enormous reduction in mortality which occurred in the preceding fifty years (figure 13).

Rubella

Rubella is a very mild infectious disease which rarely gives rise to serious complications in those infected. The need for immunization was therefore unrecognized until it was observed that congenital malformations were common in children born after a pregnancy during which the mother had contracted the infection.

Isolation of the virus in 1962 made it possible to prepare vaccines which protect against the disease, and it is now offered routinely to all girls at ages 11 to 13. Because of the possibility of pregnancy and risk to the fetus, the vaccine is not administered routinely to women of childbearing age; but it may be used in selected groups, for example in women found to be seronegative provided they are aware of the importance of avoiding pregnancy for at least two months.

The only appropriate indication of the success of vaccination would be a reduction in the frequency of malformations due to rubella; or of the abortions which are usually performed once the disease is recognized during pregnancy. It is difficult, perhaps impossible, to assess this contribution, for rubella is sometimes unrecognized, and the malformations, although characteristic of the disease, may be due to other causes.

Tetanus

Before the First World War the annual death rate from tetanus in England and Wales was 7 per million of population. The rate has declined almost continuously since that time (figure 14) and is now well below 0·5 per million.

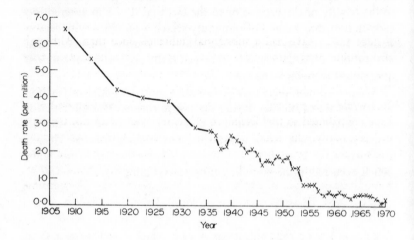

Figure 14. Tetanus. Mean annual death rate: England and Wales.

Passive immunization, in which tetanus antitoxin is given at the time of injury, has been used extensively since the First World War. However it has some serious disadvantages: it is not effective in certain cases; the protective effect is transient (about two weeks); it cannot be given in the large number of cases of minor injury which do not come to medical attention; and it is sometimes accompanied by the serious or minor reactions that may follow administration of horse serum. Active immunization by use of tetanus toxoid is effective and safe. During the Second World War it was the policy of the U.S. Armed Forces to immunize every man with tetanus toxoid on enlistment and to give a booster dose to every casualty. Among 2,750,000 wounded men there were only 12 cases of tetanus. In the British Army in the First World War, when antitoxin was used routinely after injury, the incidence of tetanus was at least 1 in 2,000 wounded. These results are not strictly comparable, but they are in accord with much other evidence that active immunization by tetanus toxoid is greatly to be preferred to passive immunization by antitoxin. National policy is now to immunize all children, and to encourage active immunization of selected groups such as patients at accident departments of hospitals, factory workers, farm workers, students and school leavers.

It is not easy to assess the contribution of immunization to the decline of mortality from tetanus shown in figure 14. It cannot have contributed before the First World War, but passive immunization is believed to have had a substantial influence since then. Although the routine active immunization of children was introduced only recently, large numbers of adults have been protected since the Second World War, including all those who have served in the armed forces. But while it is probable that both passive and active immunization have contributed to the decline of mortality, they were not the only or, necessarily, the most important influences. Other explanations (such as the disappearance of the horse from the roads) must be found for the substantial reduction of deaths before the introduction of immunization, and in recent years there has been a considerable improvement in treatment.

IMMUNIZATION IN PARTICULAR CIRCUMSTANCES

Here we are concerned with diseases against which immunization may be offered only in particular circumstances; and within this class the discussion will be restricted to conditions which occur, or are likely to occur, in Britain. On these grounds we exclude yellow fever and cholera, against which people are vaccinated only when going abroad to countries where they will be at risk. Typhoid and paratyphoid fevers are also omitted, for although a few hundred cases are notified annually in the British Isles, immunization is advised only for those going to countries with low hygienic standards, and the procedure can have had little influence on the trend of the diseases in Britain. Finally we exclude rabies and anthrax. The strict quarantine regulations make it unlikely that rabies will be seen in this country except occasionally in persons who have been infected abroad, and vaccination is recommended only for those whose occupations bring them into contact with animals in quarantine. Anthrax also is very uncommon (five cases were notified in England and Wales in 1970) and vaccination is restricted to workers exposed to risk.

The two diseases which remain are of particular interest in relation to immunization: smallpox as the infection against which vaccination was first successful, and influenza because in Britain it is probably the disease against which effective protection would now be most welcome.

Smallpox

Figure 15 shows the trend of mortality from smallpox in England and Wales since cause of death was first registered. Unfortunately, there are no reliable data for the eighteenth and earlier centuries, but the London Bills of Mortality suggest that epidemics of the disease caused a high mortality, particularly among children. In 1796 one-fifth of all deaths in London were ascribed to smallpox. Mortality declined rapidly

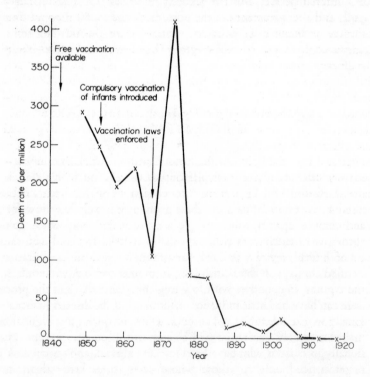

Figure 15. Smallpox. Mean annual death rate: England and Wales.

from the late nineteenth century and since about 1910 there have been relatively few deaths in the British Isles.

Vaccination was used first in 1798, made compulsory in 1852, and enforced rigorously between 1872 and 1887, when the acceptance rate for children was about 90 per cent. But parents increasingly took advantage of the conscientious objection clause, and in 1948, when compulsion ceased, less than 40 per cent of infants were being vaccinated. In 1971 it was decided that vaccination should no longer be recommended as a routine procedure in early childhood.

The way in which vaccination contributes to the control of smallpox has been a subject of controversy, broadly between those who attach importance to routine immunization of the general population and those who emphasize vaccination of all persons exposed to the disease. There is no doubt that vaccination affords a high degree of protection —probably higher than that from any other type of immunization— for a limited period. But the amount of protection declines fairly rapidly and after a number of years it is greatly reduced in a population and may be absent in an individual. It is on these grounds that some epidemiologists with great experience of smallpox are doubtful about the efficacy of the so-called eradication programmes, for they attach little importance to a claim that a high proportion of a population has been vaccinated unless it can be shown that the protection is maintained at a high level by repeated vaccination. Since this is not easily achieved in a large general population they consider it is more practical and effective to put the emphasis on the vaccination of all possible contacts. It is in the light of these considerations that in Britain it has been decided not to recommend routine vaccination in childhood, particularly since the risks from the occasional complications of the procedure are now out of proportion to the risk from smallpox itself. Vaccination is of course strongly recommended for people who may be exposed to the disease either abroad or in this country (as in the case of health service staff). The optimum procedure in countries where smallpox is still endemic is more controversial, although it would probably be agreed that routine immunization in childhood is desirable but should not lead to neglect of the even more important vaccination of contacts.

It is not easy to assess accurately the contribution that vaccination has made to the decline of mortality from smallpox (figure 15). Creighton, the historian of infectious disease, considered it useless; but this view is generally regarded as perverse and inconsistent with the evidence, which is admittedly difficult to interpret. In the light of present knowledge of the high degree of protection afforded by vaccination for a limited period, however, it seems reasonable to believe that the procedure was very effective, both in the limited period in the nineteenth century when a high proportion of children were immunized, and still more in the measures taken to prevent the spread of the disease by identification and vaccination of people exposed to smallpox.

Influenza

It is hardly necessary to emphasize the past and continuing importance of influenza as a cause of sickness and death. It is the only epidemic infectious disease which in technologically advanced countries presents today a threat comparable to that experienced in earlier centuries from diseases such as plague and typhus. Its occurrence and severity are still unpredictable, and as noted above there is no other infection from which effective protection would be more welcome, at least in developed countries.

Unfortunately this protection is not yet available. The problem is complicated by variation in the types of influenza virus, so that vaccines prepared during one epidemic may be ineffective against the next. This no doubt explains in part the conflicting evidence concerning the efficacy of influenza vaccines.

Influenza vaccine is not recommended for routine use or for the attempted control of outbreaks of influenza, but it may be offered to people with certain complaints (for example, chronic bronchitis) and to persons at special risk of exposure during an epidemic. These include health service staff and children and elderly people living in residences where the disease is likely to spread rapidly.

Since vaccination against influenza was introduced quite recently, has been restricted to certain groups, and has been shown to give only limited protection for a short time during inter-pandemic periods, it cannot so far have reduced the incidence of the disease or mortality from it.

APPRAISAL OF IMMUNIZATION

There is good reason to believe that the immunization procedures now available provide substantial protection against most of the diseases referred to above. Had these measures been in general use from the late nineteenth century it would now be impossible to assess their contribution to the decline of mortality. Almost certainly we should have overestimated it. As it is, it seems probable that immunization has had a substantial effect on the reduction of deaths from smallpox (figure 15) and diphtheria (figure 10), and more recently on the smaller problems of poliomyelitis (figure 12) and (less certainly) tetanus (figure 14). The effective procedures were too late to have much influence on two of the most important causes of death—tuberculosis and whooping cough (figures 4 and 11)—and they have had no effect at all on the trend of mortality from measles (figure 13). Indeed the reduction of mortality from the last three diseases without the assistance of immunization should remind us of the other important influences which have been operating during the period of the decline of infections—a rising standard of living, improvements in hygiene, a reduction of family size and, latterly, better treatment.

It is not possible to assess accurately the future scope of immunization in medicine but we shall refer briefly to three questions which have a bearing on it.

1. In what circumstances should a general immunization programme be discontinued? A short answer is: When the protection provided does not justify the cost and risks of immunization. Such a point may be reached when a disease becomes very uncommon; but the decision to stop vaccination can never be easy and cannot be taken solely on economic grounds. Some considerations which should influence the decision are: (a) the cost of protection (which is greater if repeated doses are required, as in the case of tetanus toxoid, than if they are not, as in the case of B.C.G.); (b) risks of vaccination (which are not inconsiderable in the case of smallpox and whooping cough, but appear to be absent in most of the other infections discussed above); and (c) the possibility of effective treatment for cases which occur.

2. What is the scope for immunization in developing countries? This is a complex question and the answer must vary according to circumstances. In many places the frequency or severity of a disease may necessitate the use of methods, even unsafe methods, not justified elsewhere. The high mortality and serious disabilities (e.g. corneal necrosis) caused by measles in West Africa justify the use of vaccines which carry some risk for malnourished children; and the risk of smallpox vaccination is acceptable where the disease is endemic.

But while circumstances vary, the principles of decision are the same as in developed countries. In each case it is desirable first to ascertain that the procedure is effective in the conditions in which it is used, and that its benefits outweigh its risks. If it is effective there are other questions to be considered: whether a general programme makes the best use of a limited number of medical and other trained workers; and how to ensure that it does not prejudice the application of other methods.

3. Are there other important diseases against which immunization is likely to become available? To the extent that this is a technical question it must be answered by the bacteriologist and virologist; our task here is to assess where the opportunities lie. In developed countries there is little doubt that the most welcome development would be effective protection against the common respiratory infections—the common cold, influenza, bronchitis and pneumonia. But there are other less common infections, such as infective hepatitis, for which immunization would also be valuable. In some less advanced countries, probably no specific measure would be more important than one which would prevent malaria. Immunization would of course be unnecessary in areas where the mosquito can be eliminated or controlled; but in large parts of Africa, for example, this control is impractical, and an effective vaccine might prove to be the only means of eliminating the disease (see Chapter 14).

FURTHER READING

CREIGHTON C. (1965) *A History of Epidemics in Britain*, 2nd Edition. Frank Cass & Co. Ltd., London.
DIXON C. W. (1962) *Smallpox*, J. & A. Churchill Ltd., London.
SPRINGETT V. H. (1971) Tuberculosis Control in Britain 1945–1970–1995. *Tubercle*, **52,** 136.

9 · SCREENING

We have seen that improvement in health hitherto has been due essentially to reduction of morbidity and mortality from infectious disease. This reduction was brought about chiefly in two ways: by preventing exposure to infection (for example from typhoid and dysentery); and by protecting the individual who might become infected, either by specific measures (such as vaccination) or by improvement in general health. The contribution of all these methods is illustrated by the history of tuberculosis. Improved housing reduced the frequency of infection; B.C.G. vaccination provided specific protection; and better nutrition increased general resistance to the disease.

However, these measures are not always successful in preventing or abating the infections, and it is then necessary to provide treatment. In some diseases, such as whooping cough and measles, the acute onset of symptoms soon brings the patient to the doctor. In others, and particularly in chronic infections such as tuberculosis, symptoms may be minimal or absent, and the patient may not be seen until the disease has reached an advanced stage. It is clearly desirable to identify these patients before they complain of symptoms, so that they can be treated and measures taken to prevent the spread of infection. This is the purpose of mass radiography of the chest for tuberculosis and routine examination of blood for venereal infection. This type of investigation, identification of a disease in its early, and if possible, pre-symptomatic stage, is referred to as 'screening'. It has been described aptly as 'the use of *quick* and *only approximate* tests or examinations to differentiate those who probably have some disorder (*especially a latent one*) from those who probably do not'. The words in italics indicate the nature and limitations of these methods. Since tests are usually applied to large population groups, they must be quick. Being quick they can be no more than approximate. And since the cases identified have not usually been recognized before the screening, the disease is likely to be latent.

The use of screening procedures is not restricted to the infections. From a public viewpoint it is essential to identify a typhoid carrier; but for the patient it may be no less important to recognize a treatable non-infectious disease, or a physical or mental handicap, of which the the effects can be mitigated by prompt services. Treatment of phenyl-ketonuria may prevent mental retardation, and provision of a hearing aid early in life can transform the outlook for a child with impaired hearing. Indeed it seems probable that in developed countries screening will have its widest application in the discovery of congenital dis-abilities (mental subnormality, partial sight, partial hearing, congenital malformations, etc.) and non-infectious illnesses (such as cancer and cardiovascular disease), both because they are now more prominent than the infections, and because the scope for prevention is relatively less.

OBLIGATIONS IN SCREENING

Screening is distinguished fundamentally from conventional medical practice, and the requirements that should be met before a screening procedure is accepted as suitable for general application arise from this distinction. It is due essentially to the difference in the position of the doctor in relation to the patient in the two cases: in the one when the patient seeks the assistance of the doctor; in the other when the doctor undertakes to identify the patient who needs his assistance.

When the patient seeks medical advice, the doctor's ethical position is relatively simple: he attempts to do his best with the knowledge and resources available to him. He cannot fairly be criticized when the state of medical knowledge does not enable him to treat effectively or even to diagnose accurately the condition about which his advice is sought; nor can he undertake in all cases to assemble the full range of facilities for investigation and treatment from which his patient might conceivably benefit.

The position is quite different in screening, when a doctor or public authority takes the initiative in investigating the possibility of illness or disability in people who have not reported signs or symptoms. There is then a presumptive undertaking, not merely that abnormality will be identified if it is present, but that those affected will derive benefit from subsequent treatment or care. This commitment is at least implicit, and except for research or the protection of public health, no-one should be expected to submit to the inconvenience of investigation or the anxieties of case finding without the prospect of medical benefit. This obligation exists even when the patient asks to be screened or to have a health examination, for his request is based on the belief that the procedure is valuable, and if it is not it is for medical people to make this known.

The ethical considerations are so fundamental to the concept of screening that it seems desirable to reflect them in its definition. Most definitions put the emphasis on the pre-symptomatic character of the investigations; that is to say they focus on their timing in relation to the stage of disease rather than on the circumstances in which they are initiated. A review of screening sponsored by the Nuffield Provincial Hospitals Trust led to the following definition: *medical investigation which does not arise from a patient's request for advice for specific complaints.* This was considered to comprise 'investigation of patients (a) who have not sought medical assistance (as with mass radiography), (b) who have sought medical assistance only for a screening test or health examination which they believe will be of value to them, and (c) who have sought assistance for a condition unrelated to a screening procedure'. This interpretation regards as the unique feature of screening the fact that investigation is initiated by the doctor rather than by the patient. It is 'the medical initiative which creates the obligation which . . . makes a strict validation procedure essential'.

There is another consideration which makes it imperative to adopt for screening a more rigorous approach than that which is followed in ordinary clinical practice: this is the scale on which a programme may be and—if it is properly validated—should be applied. The application of a new therapeutic measure is developed gradually because its use is determined by the practicing physician who assesses its merits in relation to the alternative treatments available to him. But a screening programme believed to be of value invites large scale application which may involve deployment of extensive resources at regional and national levels. Inevitably it is developed at the expense of other possible uses of health services, manpower and equipment. For example, a decision to introduce national screening for breast cancer would make heavy demands which could be met only by substantial new expenditure or by diverting staff and facilities from other work. This diversion may be justified, but it is clearly essential to show that it is before accepting breast cancer screening as suitable for widespread application. The main tasks confronting those concerned with the practice of screening are therefore to decide on an appropriate validation procedure, and to apply it to existing programmes and to new programmes before they are brought into general use.

CRITERIA FOR SCREENING

In the light of the obligations referred to above there are five requirements which it seems essential to consider carefully in relation to screening: reliability of diagnosis; effectiveness and availability of treatment; assessment of risks; operational problems; and cost and benefit. These points will be illustrated by reference to screening for breast cancer.

Reliability of diagnosis

Since diagnostic methods in screening are intended for use in large populations, they are likely to be less reliable than the methods employed in ordinary clinical practice. Moreover, failure to recognize abnormalities when they are present (false negatives) may lead to unjustified reassurance which delays diagnosis and treatment, and erroneous identification of disease (false positives) may result in unnecessary treatment which may be costly, unpleasant or even harmful. The false negative risk is far from negligible, for most screening tests have low yields and with even a small error rate the number of normals incorrectly treated may exceed the number of abnormals correctly treated.

The aim of most screening tests is of course identification of those needing further investigation, rather than precise diagnosis. But the further investigation required may expose patients to anxiety and risk. For example, in screening for breast cancer, among women considered suspect after clinical examination, nearly nine-tenths were found at biopsy not to have the disease. With clinical examination and mammography combined the proportion negative was four-fifths.

Effectiveness and availability of treatment

In ordinary clinical practice it is often necessary to use treatments whose effectiveness has not been determined fully or, sometimes, at all. In screening, however, the ethical obligations and potential costs make it essential to know that treatment is effective before a test is accepted for general application. Ideally this requires both a fairly complete picture of the natural history of the disease and a critical appraisal of treatment (the evidence available as a basis of screening for tuberculosis, for example); in practice it may be necessary to accept only an evaluation of the effects of early detection and treatment on survival.

Since it is obligatory to provide the appropriate care for those discovered to require it, the operational relationship between screening and subsequent treatment services is important. It is irresponsible to leave patients to make their own arrangements, and less than satisfactory merely to inform the patient's doctor about the results of a screening exercise in which he had no part.

Assessment of risks

The obligations of screening in relation to diagnosis and treatment apply particularly to any health hazard associated with the screening procedure itself. Regrettably it must be accepted that the ordinary practice of medicine involves risks which may arise from ignorance—as in the case of exposure to excessive radiation in the earlier treatment of tuberculosis—or because the risks, like the effectiveness of treatment, cannot be fully assessed. But when the initiative in investigation of an ostensibly healthy person is taken by the doctor, any risks must be quantified and weighed carefully in relation to the benefit from treatment. In screening for breast cancer, for example, it is not enough to believe that the risks of mammography are acceptably low; these risks must be measured accurately in relation to the frequency and type of examination and when, as with such indices, the risks fall within a range, it is the upper limit which should be used in coming to a decision about the advisability of screening. It is also necessary to take account of the stress and risk associated with biopsy, particularly since the majority of those investigated will be found not to have the disease.

Operational problems

In addition to the usual problems associated with the provision of all medical services, screening presents others which are unique to itself. One of these problems is that of public response to a service which is offered rather than requested; experience of cervical cytology suggests that the response may be least from those who have most to gain from being screened. Another problem arises from the use of staff. Screening for breast cancer, for example, makes heavy demands on the time of surgeons, radiologists and radiographers, and unless it can be shown that less expensively trained staff can be substituted, it seems unlikely that a national service could be offered. But perhaps the largest operational issue is the relation between screening and other health services. It is not difficult to imagine the unsatisfactory position which in time would result if screening programmes were developed independently, each with its own finance, administration, staff and facilities, and all separate from the main body of medical practice. In some respects the situation would be analogous to that created by malaria eradication campaigns, before it was realized that it was essential to link them with the public health services as a whole. Hence screening should not be developed in isolation but should be linked closely in its execution and follow-up with the rest of medical, diagnostic and treatment services.

Cost and benefit

Slowly, and rather reluctantly, it is becoming recognized that in time all health services will have to submit to appraisal of their cost and benefit; but in screening, for reasons discussed above, this appraisal should precede its introduction. Clearly it is not enough to know that a programme provides some benefit; before accepting it as suitable for general use we need to know how much benefit and at what risk and cost. The final decision whether to screen turns on a value judgement, but the data on which this judgement is based should be as precise as we can make them.

Again this point may be illustrated by reference to screening for breast cancer. It would not be sufficient to show that after a number of years there are fewer deaths from breast cancer among women screened than among those not screened. Ideally we need to know the increase in expectation of life which results from screening in a population of women and this benefit should be weighed in relation to the costs of screening in manpower and resources, the anxieties associated with biopsy and the risks from mammography.

APPRAISAL OF SCREENING PROCEDURES

On the basis of past experience the usefulness of some types of screening can hardly be disputed. Well established procedures include tuberculin skin tests in children, examination during pregnancy of blood pressure and of the blood for anaemia, syphilis and determination of blood group, the Coombs test on the cord blood of infants of Rh negative mothers, examination of teeth, eyesight and hearing in schoolchildren, and mass radiography of the chest. In tropical countries inspection of the blood for malaria and trypanosomiasis and of the stools for parasitic worms may be used for planning and monitoring the progress of eradication campaigns. The problems which arise in extending these methods to diseases such as breast cancer, diabetes mellitus, cervical cancer and glaucoma should not raise doubts about their usefulness in many situations.

Indeed there are grounds for thinking that a considerable extension of screening will be both possible and necessary. It will be possible because automation and electronic computers have simplified the task of analysis and interpretation of large numbers of specimens. It will be necessary because of the increasing importance of non-infectious disease, much of which can be neither prevented nor treated effectively at a late stage. Part of the answer in the case of non-infectious disease may lie in encouraging earlier reporting of symptoms. (If so it is hardly consistent to appeal to the public not to trouble the doctor about minor complaints.) But with increasing knowledge much more may depend on the use of screening procedures—biochemical, cytological, radiological, etc.—to recognize disease in the pre-symptomatic stage.

Contrary perhaps to popular belief, in technologically advanced countries screening is restricted more by lack of knowledge than by lack of resources. Where the requirements described above are met, as in the use of mass radiography for detection of tuberculosis, the method has been applied widely. The main reason for failure to employ screening for the discovery of diseases such as diabetes is that one or more of the essential requirements are not met.

Before screening can become a significant feature of medical practice, there must be a considerable advance of knowledge. This requires both clinical and laboratory research, and, even more, epidemiological investigation of experience of disease in populations: the significance of signs and symptoms; observer errors; physiological variation; interpretation of departures from 'normal'; the natural history of disease; the outcome of treatment.

Finally we should refer to multiphasic (or multiple) screening, which has been defined as 'the application of two or more screening tests in combination to large groups of people'. The procedure may also include a medical history and a clinical examination. Hence multiphasic screening is not a screening test in the usual sense, but a mechanism for executing a number of investigations at the same time. It must therefore be judged as an operational procedure.

There is clearly no objection in principle to the coordination of a number of screening tests in time and place; indeed it is desirable that the procedures should be linked operationally to one another and to medical practice as a whole. But in multiple screening as currently practised most of the tests have not been validated, and this results in two major problems. First it is difficult, if not impossible, to assess the credentials of individual tests when they are incorporated in a multiphasic programme. And secondly, if multiphasic screening in its present form comes to be regarded as an established feature of medical practice, it may well displace alternative and more effective uses of the same resources. The problem is in some respects analogous to that associated with occupational and school health services, where the unvalidated practice of routine medical examinations has diverted attention and effort from other and probably more effective methods of identifying those who need medical assistance.

FURTHER READING

Screening in Medical Care. Nuffield Provincial Hospitals Trust. Oxford University Press, Oxford (1968).

WILSON J. M. G. and JUNGNER G. (1968) *Principles and Practice of Screening for Disease*. World Health Organization, Public Health Papers 34, Geneva.

10 · MODIFICATION OF PERSONAL BEHAVIOUR

In Chapter 1 attention was drawn to the great importance of the limitation of numbers which resulted from reduction of family size, in Britain from the late nineteenth century. The change in reproductive behaviour was an indispensable condition for an improvement in human health, for without it the effectiveness of other measures would have been reduced and perhaps eliminated. This aspect of behaviour is still of enormous importance, obviously in developing countries, but also in technologically advanced societies, few of which have achieved a rate of population growth consistent with the requirements of health and welfare.

There is, however, another class of behavioural influences whose effects are even more direct: we refer to aspects of an individual's personal behaviour which may prejudice his own health. A few examples are of long standing and well recognized, as in the case of drug addiction and sexual promiscuity leading to venereal infection. But there are other behavioural influences whose widespread ill-effects are more recent (smoking, overeating and physical inactivity) or whose ill effects have only recently been sufficiently recognized (alcoholism). We shall discuss the evidence on which these habits are thought to be related to disease before considering the problems presented by their control.

SMOKING

The tobacco leaf was introduced into Europe three and a half centuries ago. In spite of claims for its medicinal value, the practice of smoking met with opposition. James I described it as 'a branch of the sin of drunkenness, which is the root of all sins' and 'a custom loathsome to the eye, hateful to the nose, harmful to the brain, dangerous to the lungs, and in the black, stinking fume thereof, nearest resembling the horrible Stygian smoke of the pit that is bottomless'. In the Swiss Canton of Berne 'the offence ranked as only one degree less odious than adultery'. But by the nineteenth century addiction to tobacco, at least by men, had become unobjectionable to most people. Its medicinal properties were discredited, but it was thought to be harmless.

This conclusion was challenged when it was reported that the proportion of smokers, and particularly of heavy smokers, was higher in male patients with cancer of the lung than in healthy men. This was the starting point for a series of inquiries into the relationship between smoking and disease. An association is now well established with cancer of the lung, chronic bronchitis, and coronary heart disease, and the evidence is suggestive in a number of other conditions. Smoking has also been shown to cause a reduction in birth weight. Much of the evidence and almost the whole of the controversy concerning the effects of smoking have been focussed on cancer of the lung and we shall limit our discussion to this disease.

The earliest investigations compared the smoking habits of patients in hospital with carcinoma of the lung with those of a control group of other hospital patients. The main findings were that the proportion of smokers was much higher among patients with the disease than among controls, and that the risk of developing carcinoma of the lung appeared to increase with increasing amounts smoked. These results have since been amply confirmed and extended by prospective studies of mortality in relation to smoking habits. These prospective studies have shown conclusively that mortality from lung cancer increases sharply with increasing amounts smoked, and, among those who have given up smoking, declines progressively with the length of time for which they have given up. The association with cigarette smoking is present only for squamous-cell and oat-cell carcinoma. The less common adenocarcinoma appears to be unrelated to smoking.

These findings are consistent with the observations that deaths from lung cancer have increased with the increasing sale of cigarettes and that in general national mortality from cancer of the lung is closely related to national tobacco consumption.

Interpretation

Before considering the objections that have been raised to the conclusion that cigarette smoking is largely responsible for lung cancer, we should refer to some apparent inconsistencies in the evidence.

(*a*) *Sex differences*. Death rates from lung cancer are about five times higher in men than in women, although male tobacco consumption is only twice as great. This difference may be explained partly by differences in smoking practices, for example in type of cigarettes, in the proportion of cigarettes smoked or in age of starting to smoke.

(*b*) *National differences*. There are a few countries (Japan, the United States and South Africa) where mortality from lung cancer is lower than would be expected from the cigarette consumption. Again there may be differences in types of tobacco consumed and smoking practices or in other influences such as atmospheric pollution.

(*c*) *Pipe and cigar smokers*. Since the amount of carcinogens in pipe and cigar smoke is at least as great as in cigarette smoke, the relatively low risk of death from lung cancer in pipe and cigar smokers would not have been expected. However there is some evidence that there are other differences between the effects of the two kinds of smoke.

Although the explanations which can be suggested for these apparent inconsistencies are not as yet fully substantiated, the inconsistencies themselves are no more than might be expected with so complex a problem, and none of them presents a serious obstacle to accepting that the association between cigarette smoking and cancer of the lung is a causal one.

Those who have challenged this have done so mainly on three grounds. In the first place it is pointed out that the statistical association does not prove that smoking causes cancer. This objection is largely met by the strength and consistency of the association, by the observation that mortality from lung cancer declines in men who give up smoking and, for those who find work on experimental animals more convincing than controlled observations in man, by the production of cancer of the lung in animals which have inhaled cigarette smoke.

A second basis of objection is that smoking produces effects that are apparently non-specific, since it is associated with increased mortality from several diseases. However there is nothing surprising in the observation that smoking, like other agents as different as alcohol, the spirochaete and psychological stress, should have multiple effects. Moreover cigarette smoke is not a single chemical agent.

Thirdly, it has been suggested that certain people are genetically predisposed both to smoke and to develop lung cancer, and thus patients owe their cancer to their genes rather than to their smoking. This hypothesis was thought to be supported by certain physical and psychological differences between smokers and non-smokers; however it is inconsistent with the large increase in death rates from lung cancer during this century, and with the rapid decrease in mortality from the disease in doctors who have stopped smoking cigarettes.

Most epidemiologists who have reviewed the evidence, taking account of the inconsistencies and the doubts which have been expressed, have no hesitation in accepting the conclusion reached in the 1971 Report of the Royal College of Physicians (Smoking and Health Now): 'The quantitative association between cigarette smoking and the development of lung cancer is most simply explained on a causal basis and no other explanation accounts for the facts.'

ALCOHOL

The history of the use of alcohol by man is almost as long as the history of man himself. Archaeologists have uncovered evidence of cereals having been used to brew fermented drinks from the very earliest times. Alcohol has been used and has also been abused since the beginning of history, to the harm of the individual and of society, and there have been many attempts to control the abuse. In the ninth century B.C. the King of Sparta decreed that all vineyards should be destroyed and the legs of drunkards cut off. In more recent times attempts have been made to enforce prohibition, with less drastic penalties, in the United States and Sweden, but with no great success. Despite heavy taxation, restrictions on the hours, places and conditions of sale, and penalties for driving with blood levels of over 80 mg per 100 ml, alcohol remains in this country the traditional and the most commonly used drug capable of producing dependence.

Alcohol is undoubtedly a major health and social problem, but it is difficult to assess its size as there is no direct measure of its effect on mortality or morbidity. An indirect and not very reliable indicator of the influence on mortality is provided by death rates attributed to cirrhosis of the liver. For example, in France adults over fifteen years of age drink the equivalent of more than 28 litres of alcohol per head per year, approximately a pint a week: in the United Kingdom the corresponding amount is about six litres a year or a tablespoon a day, to a Frenchman less than a medicinal dose. The death rate from cirrhosis of the liver in France is ten times the death rate in the United Kingdom. Mortality from cirrhosis does not appear to be increasing in Britain (it has remained at about 30 per thousand for males and 26 per thousand for females since the 1950's) but there are striking differences by social class and by occupation. The death rate for the professional classes (in social class I) is nearly three times the death rate for semi-skilled and unskilled workers (in social classes IV and V), and for hotel and innkeepers it is ten times the average for the male population as a whole.

But mortality from cirrhosis is only a small part of the death toll taken by alcohol. For example, suicides and accidental deaths are both associated with alcoholism: suicide rates are high in occupations where alcoholism is common; the suicide rate among alcoholics who have been admitted to psychiatric hospitals has been found to be eighty times higher than among men of the same ages in the general population; and in a study of men admitted for self-poisoning to hospitals in Edinburgh 39 per cent were known to be heavy drinkers. The extent to which alcohol is implicated in traffic accidents is uncertain, but 25 per cent of the drivers killed in accidents on the roads are found at postmortem to have blood alcohol levels above the statutory 80 mg per 100 ml.

It is difficult to estimate the amount of ill-health in the population directly attributable to the abuse of alcohol. This difficulty is in part related to the fact that the underlying addiction is often concealed by patients. It is also related to the difficulty of defining alcoholism, when the use of alcohol ranges from occasional social drinking to regular and heavy drinking with associated morbidity such as chronic gastritis, cirrhosis of the liver, polyneuritis and mental illness (depression, changed sexual habits, delirium tremens and Korsakow's syndrome). The World Health Organization has defined alcoholics as 'those excessive drinkers whose dependence on alcohol has attained such a degree that they show a noticeable mental disturbance or an interference with their mental and bodily health, their interpersonal relations and their smooth social and economic functioning; or who show prodromal signs of such developments'. Within the framework of this admittedly broad definition it has been estimated that there are about 350,000 alcoholics in Britain, a quarter of whom (3 per 1,000 of the adult population) show physical and mental deterioration. On any account this represents a formidable health problem.

OVER EATING

During most of man's time on earth the outstanding problem connected with food has been that there is not enough of it. It is understandable that in communities where undernutrition was widespread, obesity was commonly equated with prosperity, if not with health. In the nineteenth century the wealth of the king and princes of the Wanguana in East Africa was measured by the girth of their wives. In the Journal of the Discovery of the Source of the Nile Speke reported that from early youth the women were kept with a pot of milk to their mouths, and some of them 'were fattened to such an extent that they could not stand upright and their flesh hung down like loose stuffed puddings'.

About two thirds of the people in the world are still living in a state of chronic undernourishment, but for the first time in history there are now countries in which the opportunity to overeat is no longer confined to a trivial minority and obesity is emerging as a major health hazard. For example, in England and Wales young and middle aged men are now on the average about 14 lb heavier than men of the same age and height in the 1930's, and American males are even heavier. Life insurance statistics have provided impressive evidence of the relation between obesity and mortality. Men who are more than 25 per cent heavier than the average for their age and height have a death rate twice as high as those within five per cent of the average. The most striking differences are in respect of deaths from ischaemic heart disease, diabetes, cerebrovascular disease, chronic nephritis and accidents. Desirable standards for weight have been derived from these insurance statistics, based on the weights of men with the most favourable mortality experience. According to these standards, middle aged men in England and Wales are now on the average about 20 lb 'overweight', and there is evidence that this overweight problem begins in part in infancy—the overweight infant tends to become the overweight schoolchild and later the overweight adult.

Ischaemic heart disease is now the leading cause of death for both males and females and the death rate for males has been steadily increasing since about 1948. The increase has been most substantial for young and middle aged men, the groups that have shown the greatest increase in weight. It is reasonable to conclude in the light of all the evidence that the increase in mortality is in part attributable to the increase in weight.

PHYSICAL INACTIVITY

Men are not only becoming more obese, but with the increasing use of the motor car and the automation of industrial processes they are becoming less physically active and there is now evidence that those in sedentary jobs are at higher risk to death from ischaemic heart disease.

One of the first reports (1953) of the inverse relation between coronary disease and physical activity was based on sickness and mortality records of London Transport drivers and conductors aged 35–64 years. Drivers had more coronary disease than conductors; their disease also appeared at an earlier age and was more frequently fatal. The conclusion that this result was attributable to variation in physical activity was supported by similar findings in a comparison of the experience of government clerks and postmen, and from national statistics by a comparison of mortality in a wide range of occupations. The relationship of mortality to activity was remarkably consistent, even within the same social class. Since then a number of other epidemiological investigations have confirmed that, for men, physical activity at work appears to give considerable protection against mortality from coronary disease. One of the more recent enquiries related to a 16 year follow-up of longshore men in San Francisco, two thirds of whom (the 'active' group) were doing particularly heavy work, mainly cargo handling. The death rate from coronary heart disease was considerably lower in the active group than in the less active group. The difference was greatest for the youngest age group (35–44 years) in which the active men had a death rate only one seventh that of the less active men.

Other investigations have suggested that inactivity is associated more with sudden death from myocardial infarction than with morbidity from ischaemic heart disease, and more with occlusive coronary artery disease and myocardial scarring than with mural atheroma. They also indicate that current physical activity is probably more important than average activity throughout life. For the relationship between coronary disease and physical activity two explanations have been suggested. Exertion may lead to an increase in the coronary collateral circulation; or it may prevent intravascular clotting. (It has been shown that acceleration of plasma-clotting time after ingestion of fat is largely abolished by physical activity.) Both explanations suggest a possible accommodation between the findings described above and the large body of evidence that relates the incidence of coronary artery disease to obesity and the intake of animal fats.

THE CONTROL OF PERSONAL HABITS

The relation between personal habits and certain causes of death raises two main questions: whether the evidence is acceptable; and if it is, whether effective public action is either justified or possible.

On the first point there is no doubt about the association between, for example, smoking and lung cancer or obesity and ischaemic heart disease. But some say that without experimental confirmation a causal relationship cannot be inferred. We make three comments.

First, it is not easy to conceive of experiments which would remove all doubts. Positive results in the hamster, guinea pig or orang-outang would leave many reservations about their bearing on the aetiology of lung cancer and ischaemic heart disease in man. And human beings can scarcely be submitted to more exacting tests than those they already undertake voluntarily by smoking and overeating.

Second, experimental findings would be only *relatively* more convincing than the evidence already available. For even planned experiments are open to misinterpretation, and are more conclusive than direct observations only because they can be conducted under more controlled conditions.

Third, insistence on experimental support for conclusions which are already acceptable to many critical people may result in a large number of unnecessary deaths. In the nineteenth century the association between polluted water and cholera was regarded as sufficient reason for improving water supplies. Had experimental confirmation, or even clarification of the nature of infection been required, effective action would have been delayed by many years.

In the case of smoking the evidence is already impressive, and it would be inexcusable to delay action solely on the grounds that one day it may be even stronger. The question remains whether public intervention in personal habits is justified or likely to be effective.

On the first point the law is already clear. People are not encouraged to kill themselves; and if tobacco caused death in thirty hours instead of thirty years measures of control would be introduced very quickly. It is only because the effects are delayed, and hence are recognizable by numerical evidence rather than everyday experience, that it is possible publicly to differentiate between the effects of tobacco and the effects of narcotics.

But even if an individual is allowed to kill himself, so long as he does it slowly, it is quite another matter to permit others to create the circumstances in which he may do so inadvertently. This, essentially, is the position which results from the sale of cigarettes.

Could public intervention in private habits be effective? Again we may illustrate the possibilities with reference to tobacco. Countries must decide how far they can go in a matter of this kind, and most have already concluded that prohibition of smoking is out of the question. Nevertheless it is quite feasible to make it more difficult to smoke; for example by prohibiting all advertising and sale to young people, and by raising the cost through taxation (the last has not been very successful in the past). But on a longer view, the most effective means of control of personal habits is to create an environment in which it is easy to do what is healthy (for example to exercise) and to avoid what is harmful (to smoke). Until recently it was difficult, particularly for young men, to avoid smoking, not because they have an inborn craving for it, but because they were constantly exposed to social pressures. For the first time, perhaps, in this century, it is possible to find oneself in an environment in which the position is reserved; for example in the company of chest physicians it would require considerable determination to light up. It seems reasonable to expect that the disapproval, now exhibited particularly by socially responsible doctors, will spread, and that the time will come when a thoughtful parent will be as unwilling to set his children a bad example by smoking as by other forms of antisocial behaviour.

Finally, as the list of proscribed pleasures lengthens, it may be asked why indulgence of habits which give pleasure should be dangerous. Some people prefer sitting to walking; many like tobacco and alcohol; and nearly all enjoy food rich in certain ingredients to which they have become accustomed. Why then can they not relax, smoke, drink and eat, without risking their lives?

The most plausible answer is in terms of selection. Living organisms can adapt to profound changes, given time for those genetically ill-equipped for the new environment to die, and for those well-equipped to reproduce. But human reproduction is slow, and with the exception of alcohol the changes in personal habits to which we have referred have occurred in a very short time, mainly during the twentieth century. Eighty years ago it was exceptional for a man to smoke; it is now exceptional not to. Improved methods of food production and distribution put the temptation to overeat before large numbers of people. And physical activity has been transformed by the introduction of the motor car. In time the human body could adapt to these as to former changes; but it cannot do so rapidly, and cannot do so at all unless the effects of selection are permitted to operate. If the problem is to be resolved in this way, the death of the susceptible at an early age is the price that must be paid.

FURTHER READING

CLEAVE T. L. and CAMPBELL G. D. (1969) *Diabetes, Coronary Thrombosis and the Saccharine Disease*, 2nd Edition. John Wright & Sons Ltd., Bristol.

MORRIS J. N., HEADY J. A., RAFFLE P. A. B., ROBERTS C. G. and PARKS J. W. (1953) Coronary heart disease and physical activity of work. *Lancet*, **ii**, 1053 and 1111.

Report of the Royal College of Physicians of London (1971) *Smoking and Health Now*. Pitman Medical and Scientific Publishing Co. Ltd., London.

CONTROL OF ENVIRONMENT

11 · NUTRITION

The prescription of dietetic regimes and the treatment of nutritional disease lie in the province of clinical medicine. Our concern is with the social and community aspects of the relation between nutrition and health. The subject is extensive, and it will be dealt with in four sections. The first (*Choice of Food*) outlines some important reasons for the variation that exists in the dietetic habits of different communities. The second (*Nutritional Needs*) discusses the composition of a balanced diet and the needs of special groups (pregnant and lactating women, children and heavy manual workers). The third (*Nutrition in Britain*) describes measures introduced in this century to ensure that certain population groups get a diet more in keeping with their nutritional needs than the one they have had in the past. The final section (*Nutrition and Health*) considers the difficulty of measuring the association between diet and health, and presents some of the evidence related to the influence of nutrition upon mortality, morbidity and growth and development.

CHOICE OF FOOD

In some parts of the world malnutrition is still common; and it is not long since most people in the world lived in a state of chronic under-nourishment, with the threat of famine and death from starvation always in the background. People preoccupied with the problem of finding enough food to keep alive do not bother much about the relative proportions of the different components of their diet, and apart from the risk of acute poisoning are not much concerned with the influence of food on disease. They eat what they can get and this is determined by where they live: maritime communities live largely on fish; in the tropics the variety of naturally occurring vegetables, fruits and cereals favours vegetarianism; and people living in arctic regions depend almost entirely on the flesh and fat of seal, whale and walrus. Even in more advanced communities climate and geography have a considerable influence on diet, of which the olive oil, pasta and wine of Italy and the herrings, porridge and whisky of Scotland are examples. Moreover, in the same locality seasonal variations in availability of fruit, vegetables and animal foods are reflected in seasonal changes in diet.

Over the past century there have been unprecedented improvements in methods of producing, storing and transporting food, and climate, season and geographical position are no longer so important in determining what a community eats. In spite of these advances, food habits and standards of nutrition still vary a great deal from country to country and between different social groups. Climatic differences and religious and social customs account for some of the variation: Brahmins, Mohammedans, Jews and Catholics all have strong dietetic taboos; a Frenchman will eat snails, an Australian bushman insects, a Welshman seaweed and an Englishman corned beef and cabbage. So highly conditioned is the sense of taste that each may find his own titbit delectable and his neighbour's disgusting. But by far the greater part of the variation is due not to climatic influence or religious and social custom but to economics. This is as true at the national as at the personal level. Nations, like individuals, can have as adequate and varied a diet as they can afford.

Economic factors

Tentative assessments of the average daily calorie intake per head of the population for different countries suggest that it ranges from about 1,700 in parts of Asia, Africa, South America and the Middle East to well over 3,000 in economically advanced countries such as the United States, New Zealand, Australia, Scandinavia and the United Kingdom. In the West it is now generally agreed that in light employment a man needs only 2,750 and a woman 2,250 calories a day. The food consumption of a considerable proportion of the world's population is therefore very inadequate.

In 1956 countries with a mean annual income of less than $100 per head had an average of daily calorie intake of less than 2,000; in countries with an average income of $600 the intake was over 3,000. This is not the whole of the story; the energy content of a diet is a very incomplete measure of its nutritional value, and with increasing national income, consumption of carbohydrate increases much less rapidly than consumption of the more expensive and nutritionally more valuable proteins and fats.

There is also plenty of evidence that within a country variation in family income has a profound influence on dietetic habits. During the period 1932–35, Boyd-Orr collected information about the food purchases and incomes of 1,152 families, mostly living in the industrial north of England. Families with a per capita income of £2·25 or more per week consumed five times the amount of fresh milk and fish, more than three times the amount of butter and eggs and twice the amount of meat consumed by those living on income of less than 50p per head per week. In contrast, the poorest families ate three times the amount of margarine.

NUTRITIONAL NEEDS

Nutritional needs are a matter, first of energy requirements—which is largely a question of the quantity of food consumed—and second, of the relative proportions of the different nutrients needed—which is more a question of the quality or composition of the diet. These two aspects of the problem will be considered separately.

Energy requirements

It has been estimated that the requirement per head for the population of the United Kingdom is about 2,500 calories a day. In many parts of the world the amount of food consumed is insufficient to provide even 2,000 calories a day, yet death from starvation is not common. The explanation of this paradox lies in the fact that estimates of calorie needs are based on well nourished persons. When food intake is inadequate, body weight, basal metabolism and capacity for physical and mental exertion are all greatly reduced; life is maintained at a lower level and death due to or accelerated by nutritional disease is more common.

The calorie needs of children and adolescents are very high in relation to their size, partly because of the requirements of growth, and partly because of their intense physical activity. It is a common observation that adolescents usually eat much more than their parents. Girls have their maximum need at about 14, when it is 40 per cent higher than that of women in sedentary employment. The need of boys rises steadily until they are about 17, when it is 60 per cent higher than that of men in sedentary employment.

During the first half of pregnancy a woman's requirements are not greatly increased; but in the second half her basal metabolic rate may be more than 20 per cent higher than it was before the pregnancy began, and during lactation she needs an extra 500 calories a day.

A balanced diet

Throughout the world the cheapest foods are usually those which consist principally of starch (rice, potatoes, wheat, maize, oats and rye) and the standard of living of families, communities or countries can be gauged by the amount of starch in their diets. Cereals and potatoes provide about one-third of the calorie value of food consumed in the United States, Canada, New Zealand, Switzerland, Sweden and the United Kingdom, whereas they provide nearly nine-tenths of the calories in China, India, South East Asia and much of Africa. A diet consisting almost entirely of carbohydrates has serious disadvantages: it is bulky and satisfies hunger before it has met energy requirements (7 lb of potatoes and a 2 lb loaf each provide only a little over 2,000 calories); and because it is often short of essential nutrients it is likely to give rise to deficiency disease.

Weight for weight fats have more than twice the calorie value of carbohydrates and therefore play an important part in reducing the bulk of the diet of persons with heavy energy demands (manual workers, adolescents and persons living in very cold climates). For most people fatty foods help to make a diet more palatable and they are also the principal source of fat-soluble vitamins.

The proteins in meat, milk, eggs and cheese contain all the essential amino acids necessary for growth and health which cannot be synthesized in the body; but most vegetables and cereals are deficient in one or more of them. However, animal proteins can safely be dispensed with if the diet includes a reasonable variety of vegetable foods.

More than twenty 'accessory food factors' are now recognized and many have been synthesized. Much of the knowledge about the part they play in growth, development and maintenance of health has been acquired by means of animal experiment and cannot be applied directly to the problem of nutritional needs in man. But it is known that a diet deficient in vitamin C causes scurvy and one deficient in vitamin D, calcium and phosphorus gives rise to rickets or osteomalacia. We also know that beri-beri is associated with lack of thiamine, pellagra with lack of nicotinic acid and pernicious anaemia with lack of vitamin B_{12}.

For the rest, knowledge of the relation between vitamins and growth and health in man is still incomplete. From the social viewpoint, however, three important facts stand out: most foodstuffs rich in vitamins are also relatively expensive (dairy produce, meat, eggs and fruit); there is seasonal variation of vitamin intake; and some modern methods of food handling seriously impair nutritive value by substantially reducing vitamin content (refining flour and sugar, polishing rice, canning vegetables and fruit, etc.).

Many mineral substances are also essential to life. They include calcium, phosphorus, sodium, potassium, magnesium, sulphur, chlorine, iron, iodine, copper, cobalt, fluorine, manganese and zinc. Most of them are required in such small quantities, however, that, with the important exceptions of calcium and iron, almost any diet provides enough to meet the body's needs. In childhood, pregnancy and during lactation much more calcium is required than at other times. The transfer of iron to the fetus during pregnancy or loss from haemorrhage at delivery or menstruation is a common cause of anaemia. Dairy produce and bread are the principal natural sources of calcium and meat and green vegetables of iron. Hence calcium and iron deficiencies are likely to be associated with poverty and are commonest in infancy, childhood, during or after childbearing and in old age.

NUTRITION IN BRITAIN

As recently as the eighteenth century death from starvation was common in bad harvest years in Britain. Today the position is very different. The diet of even the poorest members of the community is nearly always adequate in calorific value, and it is not often grossly deficient in any of the essential nutrients. Frank deficiency disease has become a clinical rarity and death from starvation is almost unknown. A considerable part of this remarkable improvement has taken place since the beginning of the twentieth century. To some extent this has been brought about by a deliberate if not very precisely planned nutritional policy. The reasons for major social changes are always complex but four broad influences are discernible.

Undernourishment in children

The first influence was a growing public awareness in the early years of this present century of a great deal of undernourishment among poor children. Such children had always been short of food, but for the first time evidence of the extent and importance of this social evil began to accumulate. After the introduction of compulsory education, teachers began to draw attention to the fact that many of the children now required to attend school were too sick and hungry to benefit much from the teaching offered. This observation was substantiated in the study by Seebohm Rowntree of the conditions under which the poor were living in York and confirmed by the report of the Inter-Departmental Committee on Physical Deterioration (1904), a Committee appointed after the Director-General of the Army Medical Service had revealed that between 40 and 60 per cent of the young men presenting themselves for military service at the time of the South African War had been rejected on medical grounds. The Committee produced a great deal of evidence about the amount of malnutrition in children and concluded that probably one-third of the poorer children in the country were not getting enough to eat. As a result of this and similar reports a national policy of feeding necessitous children at school was initiated with the Education (Provision of Meals) Act, 1906.

The science of nutrition

A second influence was the impact upon public opinion of the advances made in the science of nutrition in the early decades of this century. In the nineteenth century scientific interest had been focussed upon fats, proteins and carbohydrates and the amount of energy they provided. It was generally believed that a diet was adequate if it satisfied hunger and provided enough calories to meet the body's energy needs. In the late nineteenth and early twentieth centuries the animal experiments of Eijkman, Gowland Hopkins and others, showed that an adequate diet was more than a matter of calorific value of the three basic nutrients. Attention was now directed towards the quality of foodstuffs as distinct from their quantity, and 'vitamin' became a household word. In the late 1920s the practical implications of this knowledge were made clear by the demonstration that a little extra milk each day could produce a striking acceleration in the growth rate of schoolchildren. Public interest was aroused, the whole question of minimum dietetic requirements in relation to age and occupation came under review and detailed recommendations were made by various bodies.

Dietary surveys left no doubt that by the recommended standards many people were living on very inadequate diets. The relation between undernourishment and poverty was underlined by the work of Boyd Orr. He pointed out that the poorest families are usually the largest families, and that the larger a family the less money there is per head to spend on the relatively expensive protective foods, in particular dairy produce. The growth of the school meals service during the inter-war years, the distribution of milk to necessitous and undernourished schoolchildren in the 1920s (extended in 1934 to all schoolchildren), the provision of free or cheap milk to expectant and nursing mothers and pre-school children, and the emphasis placed by the growing maternity and child welfare movement upon infant and maternal nutrition, can all be traced to the advances in the science of nutrition.

The impact of war

A third influence on the improvement in nutritional status was, paradoxically, the shortage of food during the two world wars. Since the last quarter of the nineteenth century Britain has become progressively more dependent upon imported foodstuffs to feed the expanding population. (At the present time we grow less than half our food.) Towards the end of the 1914–18 war German submarines had destroyed so much shipping that food imports were reduced to a dangerously low level. A national food policy was introduced. Home production of essential foodstuffs was stepped up; measures were taken to control the price and distribution of many foods; and sugar, meat, milk, butter and margarine were rationed. The lessons learned were of great service twenty years later when at the beginning of the second world war a Ministry of Food was at once established. The aim of the Ministry was to encourage maximum home production and to ensure as far as possible that food was distributed according to need, with priority for nutritionally vulnerable groups such as children and expectant and nursing mothers. Essential foodstuffs were rationed, and their price controlled by subsidies. The 'Milk in Schools' scheme was extended and extra milk and cod liver oil and fruit juices were made available to all expectant mothers and children under five. Factories employing more than 200 workers were required to provide a canteen service, and British Restaurants, serving substantial meals at cost price, were set up to meet the needs of workers who did not have access to a canteen. Margarine was fortified with vitamins A and D and the nutritional value of wheat flour was raised by increasing the extraction rate and adding calcium carbonate.

National food policy was so successful that it has been claimed, with some justification, that by 1944 the working class diet was nutritionally more satisfactory than at any time before. This improvement has been maintained.

Rise in standard of living

A fourth and probably the most important influence has been a substantial improvement in the standard of living. There are some uncertainties about the trend of living standards in the early years of the Industrial Revolution, but there is no doubt that they were rising by the mid nineteenth century and have continued to improve, with interruptions, to the present day. The effects of better living standards are multiple, but in relation to health probably none is more important than the greater expenditure on food. In some well-to-do population groups this expenditure may now be excessive, but for most people its effects have been wholly beneficial. Probably for the first time in man's history there are large populations which are adequately fed.

NUTRITION AND HEALTH

A diet grossly deficient in calories leads to loss of weight, impaired physical efficiency and eventually to death from starvation. A diet grossly deficient in certain essential nutrients results in readily recognizable clinical diseases (scurvy, rickets, keratomalacia, beri-beri, pellagra, etc.). But, as yet, little is known about the long-term effects of diets moderately deficient in calories or essential nutrients, and the subtler questions of the precise relation between nutrition and rate of growth, resistance to infection, fertility and mental performance remain for the most part unanswered.

Knowledge from animal experiments

From laboratory experiments a great deal more is known about the dietetic needs of the rat, the mouse and the guinea pig than about nutritional needs and deficiency disease in man. For example, if female rats are deprived of vitamin E (the fat-soluble tocopherols in which wheat-germ oil is particularly rich) their pregnancies terminate with fetal death at about the end of the first third of gestation. In rabbits vitamin E deficiency leads to a primary dystrophy of the voluntary muscles. Clinicians applied this knowledge with enthusiasm to their patients although there was no convincing evidence either that vitamin E deficiency occurs naturally in man or that vitamin E used therapeutically has any effect upon habitual abortion or progressive muscular dystrophy. However, the relation between diet and scurvy, rickets, keratomalacia, beri-beri and pellagra is clear enough, and these diseases are still a common cause of disability and premature death in many parts of the world. Because whole wheat has been our staple cereal for centuries, the incidence of the vitamin B complex deficiency diseases has never been high, but as we have noted, scurvy and rickets were common until the end of the nineteenth century. Today both are rare, although scurvy is still sometimes found in neglected old people and rickets has appeared among children of immigrants.

Dietetic supplements

The value of the appropriate nutritional supplement in clinically recognizable cases of deficiency disease is not in doubt. With that exception it is very difficult to make direct observations under reasonably controlled conditions of the effect of inadequate feeding upon health in man. Useful information has been obtained about vitamin A and vitamin C requirements by depriving human volunteers under controlled laboratory conditions. But of greater interest, because of their wider implications, have been observations on the effect of supplementing the diet of selected population groups thought to be taking an inadequate diet. One of the earliest and most convincing of these experiments was carried out by Corry Mann in 1926. He divided boys in an industrial school into a number of comparable groups. One group was given the usual school diet; the other groups were given various supplements (milk, butter, margarine, sugar, caseinogen, water cress). At the end of twelve months boys on the ordinary diet were on the average 1·84 inches taller and 3·85 lb heavier; boys receiving extra milk were 2·63 inches taller and 6·98 lb heavier (the only other group who approached their rate of growth was the one receiving extra butter). Children and adolescents today are considerably taller and heavier for their age than at the beginning of the century. Corry Mann's observations, and many others suggest that most of this improvement is probably due to greater consumption (and more equitable distribution) of protective foods, particularly of dairy produce.

There have been a few convincing observations on the effect of inadequate nutrition in pregnancy. The evidence suggests that an unsatisfactory diet may add appreciably to the risk of toxaemia, premature birth, stillbirth and neonatal death. The Ministry of Health claimed at the end of the war that 'the national provision of milk and vitamin supplements ... has probably done more than any other factor to promote the health of expectant mothers and young children during the war, and this scheme, together with rationing and the greatly improved nutritional qualities of the national loaf, has contributed to the gradual decline in maternal, neonatal and infant mortality and stillbirth rates, so noteworthy in the last five years'.

FURTHER READING

DRUMMOND J. C. and WILBRAHAM A. (1957) *The Englishman's Food.* Jonathan Cape, London.
ORR J. B. (1936) *Food, Health and Income.* Macmillan and Co., London.

12 · FOOD-BORNE DISEASE

An adequate and well-balanced diet is necessary for health, but food is also the source of much ill-health. The gastrointestinal tract is the usual portal of entry for many infectious and parasitic organisms, and food-stuffs readily become contaminated through human, insect and other intermediaries. In addition, a number of organisms pathogenic to man are natural pathogens of domestic animals and of rats and mice; and toxic chemicals may be introduced into food accidentally or deliberately at any stage between production and consumption.

Control of the cleanliness and composition of food is clearly important, but it is more complex and difficult than ensuring a safe water supply. Once the danger to the community of faecal contamination of drinking water has been recognized control can be left to engineers and bacteriologists, for it demands little or no cooperation from the consumer. But the effectiveness of legislation concerned with the conditions under which food is prepared, stored, distributed and eaten must always depend to some extent upon the individual.

Detailed study of the many ways in which food may become contaminated with pathogenic microorganisms lies in the domain of bacteriology; and the problems associated with the introduction of chemicals into food are primarily a matter for pharmacologists and toxicologists. We shall limit our discussion in this chapter to brief accounts of some of the major sources of contamination with micro-organisms and toxic chemicals and to a summary of the evolution and present status of control of those hazards.

CONTAMINATION WITH MICROORGANISMS

Food contaminated with microorganisms may lead either to food
poisoning or to transmission of infectious disease. Bacteriologically
these two hazards overlap; but in clinical and public health practice it
is useful to treat them as separate entities.

Food poisoning

Clinically, food poisoning is characterized by an acute gastroenteritis
of abrupt onset and short ingestion to onset period affecting several
and sometimes many people simultaneously. The majority of outbreaks are due to the presence of the salmonella group of organisms,
usually in processed and made up meat (shepherd's pie, cold ham and
bacon, pork pies, etc.) and in milk and eggs (particularly duck eggs)
and their products, but occasionally in fish, fruit and vegetables. The
organisms multiply readily in cooked and uncooked food kept at
room temperature, and from twelve to eighteen hours after they are
ingested give rise to a short-lived but prostrating gastroenteritis. Apart
from the salmonellae, the only common causes of bacterial food
poisoning are certain strains of Staphylococcus aureus and Clostridium
Welchii. These organisms also proliferate in cooked or uncooked food
stored at ordinary temperatures, but growth is inhibited at refrigerator
temperatures. The food poisoning is due to their toxins. These toxins
are heat-stable, so that infected food may give rise to poisoning even
after it has been cooked or reheated. Another well-known but fortunately rare cause of bacterial food poisoning is Clostridium botulinum,
a soil anaerobe which sometimes finds its way into processed meats,
fish products and canned and bottled foods. This organism produces
a powerful neurotoxin which has caused death from respiratory
paralysis in about half the reported cases.

The spread of communal feeding in factory canteen, school dining
room and restaurant has led to a considerable increase in the number
of reported outbreaks of food poisoning in recent years.

Transmission of infectious disease

Many bacterial and some viral and parasitic diseases are transmitted
by contaminated food. Sometimes the food is infected at source

(bovine tuberculosis and brucellosis). More often the pathogen is introduced into the food because it has been handled by someone carrying the infection (dysentery, typhoid and paratyphoid) or it has come into contact with contaminated water. The typhoid epidemic in Aberdeen, 1964, was traced to corned beef, tins of which had been cooled in contaminated water after sterilization, and the bacteria had entered through minor defects in the seams and possibly through pin holes in the tin plate itself.

In the past, milk was probably the most important cause of food-borne disease. It forms an excellent culture medium for many pathogens and has frequently been responsible for outbreaks of dysentery, typhoid and paratyphoid fever, streptococcal sore throat and infantile gastroenteritis, as well as for bone, joint and glandular tuberculosis and brucellosis. Occasionally it causes outbreaks of scarlet fever, diphtheria and staphylococcal infection. The struggle to free Britain from bovine tuberculosis was protracted and in this matter we lagged behind the United States, Canada and Scandinavia. Abdominal tuberculosis in children under 15 has nearly always been due to infected milk, so mortality from that condition provides a good index of the amount of bovine tuberculosis. In 1921 the death rate in England and Wales was 94 per million children under 15; today, children in Britain very rarely die from abdominal tuberculosis, for nearly all our milk is pasteurized and dairy herds are tuberculin negative.

Mortality from intestinal infectious diseases is today less than one-fiftieth of its level at the beginning of the century. Not all this improvement is due to cleaner food: typhoid fever is commonly water-borne; a great deal of dysentery is spread by direct contact; and in recent years more effective therapy has made a contribution. However, much of the improvement is undoubtedly due to statutory control of cleanliness of food.

Young children are particularly susceptible to bowel infection from contaminated milk. In 1908 the Medical Officer of Health for Croydon reported that the infant mortality rate from diarrhoea was 8 per 1,000 for breast fed children, 65 for children fed on fresh cows' milk and 129 for children fed on condensed milk. In 1911 infant mortality from diarrhoea in England and Wales was 36; in 1970 infant mortality from all causes was only 18 and mortality from enteritis was 0·3.

CHEMICAL CONTAMINATION

A steady rise in real wages has brought an increasing demand for a
varied and attractive diet. At the same time, more than half of our
food is imported and three-quarters of the population live in large
towns. These factors have led to an unprecedented increase in the
quantity and variety of chemicals used in the production, preparation,
preservation and presentation of food. During these processes, toxic
chemicals may get into the food by accident or they may be introduced
deliberately.

Accidental contamination

Until recently, accidental contamination of food on a large scale was
uncommon. An often quoted example (also referred to in another
context) is the epidemic of lead poisoning in the eighteenth century
due to the use of lead pipes, containers and presses in the preparation
of Devonshire cider. Today the hazard of accidental contamination is
less obvious and more widespread. In the first place harmful chemicals
may find their way into foodstuffs during production; many are used
in agriculture to protect plants against animal, insect and fungal pests.
The Working Party on Toxic Chemicals in Agriculture and Residues
in Foods set up by the Ministry of Agriculture, Fisheries and Food in
1963 listed more than a hundred preparations, some of them powerful
poisons, that present a serious hazard to agricultural workers handling
them. In addition, the antibiotics and hormones used in animal
husbandry are not without danger. For example, penicillin in the milk
of cows treated for mastitis may give rise to unpleasant reactions in
sensitized persons and may lead to sensitization in others. Harmful
chemicals may also be introduced accidentally into food during
processing and storage. Disinfectants, catalysts and bleaching and
clarifying agents are all widely used in the food industry and the
possibility of contamination of canned food with metals, particularly
zinc and lead, is a matter for concern.

Since the alarming epidemic of irreversible and gross damage to
the nervous system of people living around the estuaries of Minamata
and Niiagatu in Japan, there has been much concern about the pollution
of fishing waters with industrial effluents containing mercury. The
rising levels of methyl mercury found in the fish in certain lakes in
Sweden and North America has increased that concern.

Chemical manipulation

In the eighteenth and nineteenth centuries alum, chalk and even bone ash ('the charnel bones of the dead are raked to add filthiness to the food of the living') were added to flour to give it bulk; lead preparations were used to sweeten and clear cheap wines of sediment; infusions of oak chips were added to diluted sulphuric acid and sold as vinegar; and poisonous mixtures of sulphuric acid, turpentine and alum were sold as gin. Fraudulent adulteration of food is no longer common, but chemical manipulation of food to preserve and 'improve' it is widespread and difficult to control. Recognized practices include the addition of antioxidants, moisture retaining agents and surface protections to preserve food; sweeteners, acidifiers and spices to heighten flavour; dyes, bleaching agents, clarifiers and glazes to improve appearance; and emulsifiers, thickeners and tenderisers to improve consistency. During the course of a year we are now each consuming with our food about three pounds of chemical substances which are not natural constituents of that food and the amount is increasing. It must be remembered, however, that the nutrition of the malnourished and rapidly expanding world population is becoming more and more dependent on pesticides, antibiotics, hormones and chemical methods of food preservation.

Services for the control of food-borne disease

As far back as records go there have been prosecutions for selling adulterated foods. But the casual prosecution of a few of the worst offenders made little mark upon the problem and the evil remained practically unabated until the middle of the nineteenth century. Public control was impossible so long as there were no local authorities to operate the machinery of the law and no way of defining purity except in terms of taste, smell and appearance.

By the eighteenth century a modification of Robert Boyle's hydrometer was in fairly general use for the praiseworthy purpose of keeping the water out of the wine, and a few simple tests had been devised to detect and measure some of the commoner inorganic poisons that found their way into food. The turning point was the campaign launched by the *Lancet* in the middle of the nineteenth century, when it set up its own 'Analytical and Sanitary Commission'. Nearly 3,000 wholesale and retail purveyors of food were found guilty of selling grossly adulterated products and their names were published in the columns of the Journal. The first Food and Drugs Act (1860) was the direct result of the public outcry.

Today the control of the purity and cleanliness of food is largely a local authority responsibility. Most of the measures are to be found in the Food and Drugs Act, 1955, and in regulations made under that Act. They include food sampling for chemical analysis, and the routine inspection of meat, milk and other foods for the presence of pathogens. An authorized officer of the local authority may at all reasonable times examine food intended for human consumption, and if it appears unfit he may seize it and a magistrate will decide what further action should be taken. Minimum standards are laid down for the construction, equipment and cleanliness of premises on which food is handled, prepared or processed and particular attention is paid to the inspection of dairies and the control of persons with access to milk.

Medical practitioners have an important role to play in the control of food-borne disease. Food poisoning, enteric fever and dysentery are compulsorily notifiable and the doctor in charge of a suspected case of food poisoning should retain for bacteriological examination a specimen of faeces or vomit, and if possible, the remains of the suspected meal.

The problem of controlling chemical additives is a formidable one. Tests for general toxicity are expensive and time consuming. Tests for long-term toxic effects, and in particular for carcinogenicity, are even more expensive, take much longer and can never be entirely conclusive. Nevertheless there is clear need for such tests. For example nitrosamines, which are highly carcinogenic, have been found in foodstuffs intended for human consumption, and it is known that the nitrates traditionally used to smoke fish can react with certain amines produced in fish to form nitrosamines. With the increasing volume of international food traffic, the problem has become worldwide and a joint committee of the Food and Agricultural organization and the World Health Organization is actively concerned with international standards.

13 · WATER-BORNE DISEASE

Without water there can be no life. The need for it directs the wanderings of nomadic tribes and determines the site and size of agricultural communities. Navigable rivers have been the cradles of civilization and population growth has often been limited by the extent to which arid but potentially fertile land bordering rivers can be irrigated. The Tigris and the Euphrates watered Babylonian civilization and Egypt is still dependent upon the Nile.

For the maintenance of health, particularly in congested urban communities, a good supply of clean water is needed. If the supply is inadequate for personal and public hygiene (bathing, washing clothes and domestic utensils, cleaning streets and removing sewage and trade effluents) the spread of diseases associated with domestic and communal squalor is encouraged; and if it is not protected against contamination with pathogenic organisms and toxic substances, outbreaks of water-borne disease are likely to occur.

AN ADEQUATE WATER SUPPLY

The rate at which water is used in modern towns varies considerably from town to town and from country to country. Most big cities in Great Britain use about 60 gallons per head per day; in the cities of the United States the consumption is twice that amount. Although it is conventional to define the amount of water used in terms of consumption per head, in large industrial towns less than half the total quantity

consumed is used for domestic purposes; the rest is needed for municipal purposes (removal of sewage, cleansing of streets, fire-fighting and
supplying public baths and ornamental waters) and for industry
(about 200,000 gallons are used in the manufacture of one motor car).

In many parts of the world the direct storage of rain in cisterns and
tanks is still a common method of ensuring a minimum supply of
water, but in Great Britain, except in a few isolated communities, this
source is no longer relied upon. Urban needs are met by water from
natural and artificial lakes in upland districts and from rivers and
underground sources. Upland water is usually soft (free from calcium
and magnesium salts in solution), underground water is commonly
hard, and river water before it is purified is often grossly polluted.

A SAFE WATER SUPPLY

A safe water supply is more important to the health of a population
than any drug in the Pharmacopoeia, yet in many parts of the world it
remains a pressing health need.

Contamination with pathogenic organisms

With few exceptions (guinea worm infestation is one), the major water-
borne diseases are transmitted by contamination of water supplies with
infected human faeces or urine, so for practical purposes a safe water
supply is one protected from contact with human excreta and treated
to destroy any pathogenic organisms inadvertently introduced.

Cholera is the outstanding example of a major epidemic disease
spread through faecal contamination of drinking water, although it can
also be transmitted by infected food and by direct contact. It is a disease
of great historical interest. For centuries it has been endemic in Bengal.
In the nineteenth century it became pandemic and on six occasions
reached Europe, where it gave rise to devastating epidemics. In 1831,
1848, 1853, and 1865 explosive outbreaks of the disease in the overcrowded, unsanitary and rapidly expanding industrial towns of
England and Wales caused great public alarm and helped the public
health movement to gather momentum. During the epidemic of
1848 alone 53,000 deaths were attributed to cholera and a further
19,000 to diarrhoea. John Snow traced the spread of infection to the
contamination of drinking water by the excreta of cholera patients

and suggested that the disease might be due to invisible living organisms. In 1883, thirtyfour years later, Koch discovered the cholera vibrio.

Typhoid fever is the only other major water-borne infectious disease of which we in England and Wales have had any great experience. In 1875 the death rate from typhoid was 370 per million; in 1905 it was 115 and today it is less than 1 per ten million. When the disease was common, as it still is in many parts of the world, it was due to wholesale pollution of drinking water with the faeces and urine of cases and of carriers. From two to five per cent of patients continue to excrete the organism for months and sometimes for years after they have recovered from the disease; and although the organism does not multiply it can remain alive in water for long periods. In countries with high standards of sanitation and water purification localized outbreaks still occur. They may be due to accidental pollution of the water supply, as in Croydon in 1937, when there was a carrier in the gang of men employed to clean out a deep well. More commonly they are due to contamination of food, in particular of milk and its products, and of shellfish and canned meats.

Other water-borne diseases of international importance include amoebic dysentery (common in Africa, India, South America and the Far East) and schistosomiasis (widespread in Africa and the Far East). Between them these two water-borne diseases are responsible for an enormous amount of ill-health.

Even in countries with stringent regulations to protect and purify drinking water, accidental gross contamination can still occur. In 1926 because of a faulty mains connection Poplar was for a short time supplied with unpurified river water, and in 1936 a chalk well in Surrey became polluted by seepage from an unsuspected fracture in a nearby sewer. Characteristic localized explosive outbreaks of non-specific diarrhoea and vomiting resulted.

The virus of poliomyelitis is excreted in the faeces of patients and carried and can be isolated in sewage effluents during, and for some time after, an epidemic; but modern methods of water purification kill the virus and drinking water has not been implicated in the epidemic spread of the disease.

Contamination with toxic substances

Deep well water can cause diarrhoea when it is heavily impregnated with soluble sulphates; a suspension of microscopic particles of sand or mica, can also cause diarrhoea; and very occasionally minute quantities of arsenic find their way into upland water from sheep dip and weed killer applied in the catchment area.

Lead pipes were commonly used for domestic cold water systems. Some waters contain salts which react with the lead in such a way that the inside of the pipes become lined with insoluble compounds. Certain waters, however, are plumbo-solvent and concentrations of lead as low as one part per million have been known to cause symptoms of lead poisoning. Upland waters from peaty districts are particularly dangerous because of their acidity. An outbreak of chronic lead poisoning from this cause was reported in Sheffield as long ago as 1885. To reduce plumbo-solvency, lime or sodium silicate is added to water supplies of this type.

Protection of supplies

The problem of preventing epidemic water-borne disease resolves itself largely into a matter, first of purifying the domestic water supply, and seond, of providing an efficient sewage disposal system.

With appropriate treatment even grossly polluted water can be made safe. Many large towns use as their main sources of water rivers heavily contaminated with sewage effluents from upstream towns, and with untreated waste from isolated factories, farms and houses on their banks. (London drinks the sewage effluents of Maidenhead, Reading and Oxford.)

In the towns of this country water carriage systems are almost universally employed to remove domestic discharges and trade effluents from the neighbourhood of purified water supplies. Gross solids are screened from the sewage and most of the remaining solid matter is allowed to separate out as sludge in special tanks. Finally the organic matter in the tank liquor is biologically oxidized into simpler and less offensive compounds and the resulting effluent is discharged into neighbouring streams or rivers. However, the final effluent is still contaminated with coliform organisms, and pathogens can often be isolated from it.

APPRAISAL OF SERVICES

The introduction into Great Britain of efficient water purification and sewage disposal schemes in the second half of the nineteenth century undoubtedly made an important contribution to the decline in mortality at that time. It is impossible now to assess the extent of that contribution, but while water-borne disease is still a leading cause of death and disability over much of the world, in this country cholera has disappeared from the epidemiological scene and mortality from typhoid fever, dysentery and non-specific gastroenteritis has declined dramatically. Today the safety of the water supply is so much taken for granted that we remember the importance of the services only on the rare occasions when they break down. Three important problems remain: the pollution of coasts and rivers with sewage effluents and trade wastes; the question of fluoridation of water supplies; and the question of the relation between softness of water supplies and mortality from ischaemic heart disease.

As towns have become cleaner coasts and rivers have become progressively more filthy. Almost all our coastal holiday towns persist in the nasty habit of pouring their largely untreated sewage directly into the sea. A Medical Research Council Memorandum reported in 1959 that many samples of sea water contained thousands of coliform organisms per 100 ml, and counts of over 100,000 were recorded. (When the coliform count in water from a public supply rises much above 10 per 100 ml an outbreak of water-borne disease is likely.) However, there is little or no evidence that bathing in polluted sea-water gives rise to bowel infection or to poliomyelitis and objections to that practice rest on aesthetic grounds and the temperature of the water surrounding the British Isles.

River pollution is more serious. Rivers have a strong propensity to purify themselves by oxidizing organic contaminants, but their ability to do this is limited. As the amount of sewage effluent and industrial waste (acids, alkalis, phenols, cyanides) poured into them mounts, a point is reached beyond which purification no longer takes place. Fish die, putrefactive bacteria multiply and the water cannot be made safe for domestic use even after extensive treatment. Eighty years of exhortation, special reports, Royal Commissions and legislation have slowed down this unsavoury trend and in some instances even reversed it—the Thames, for instance, is now much cleaner than is was in the 1960's.

For a long time it has been known that drinking water containing four or more parts per million of fluoride produces a permanent mottling of dental enamel in children. More recently it has been observed that children who have been drinking water containing fluorides at concentrations below that which causes mottling show a relative immunity to dental caries. In 1944 it was reported that the incidence of dental caries among 12-year-old children in South Shields (1·4 parts of fluoride per million) was 45 per cent less than among children of the same age and comparable social status in North Shields (0·25 parts per million). All available evidence indicated that fluorides at this concentration are harmless to health, so controlled experiments were carried out in the United States, in Canada and more recently in the United Kingdom (in Anglesey, Watford and Kilmarnock) to assess the effect of artificial fluoridation to the level of one part per million. In each experimental area there was a striking improvement in the teeth of young children. In the British studies there was a sixtysix per cent reduction in caries among three year old children born after the introduction of fluoridation. There has however been considerable opposition from a small but vocal minority to the proposal that fluoridation of water supplies should become general. The opposition was so effective in Kilmarnock (one of the towns included in the British controlled experiment) that in 1962, six years after the introduction of fluoridation, it was discontinued. The amount of decay in the children's teeth in that Scottish burgh has now risen again to pre-fluoridation levels.

Finally, the association between mortality from coronary disease and the softness of local water supplies must be mentioned. In Britain, Japan, the United States, Sweden and some other countries, areas with a hard water supply appear to have lower death rates from cardio-vascular disease (in particular from ischaemic heart disease) than areas with soft water. If the cardiovascular disease death rate for men aged 45–64 in England and Wales as a whole were as low as in towns with very hard water supplies, there would be 8,000 fewer deaths each year. But rainfall, latitude and social factors as well as water calcium are associated with cardiovascular mortality, and all are associated with one another. This is an example of the need for caution in interpreting correlation as evidence of causation. The relationship may perhaps be causal (in the sense that metal or other contaminants in soft waters in some way increase the risk of death from coronary disease or the mineral content of hard waters in some way protects against it). But much more research is needed (including research on the technical problems of increasing water hardness) before a controlled trial of hardening soft water supplies, analogous with the fluoridation trials, would be justified.

FURTHER READING

Snow, John (1855) *On Mode of Communication of Cholera*. John Churchill, London. Reprinted (1965) as *Snow on Cholera*. Hafner, New York and London.

Department of Health and Social Security, etc. (1969) Reports on Public Health and Medical Subjects No. 122, *The Fluoridation Studies in the United Kingdom and the Results Achieved after Eleven Years*. H.M.S.O., London.

14 · ANIMAL-BORNE DISEASE

It is difficult to exaggerate the importance of other animals (arthropods as well as vertebrates) as reservoirs and transmitters of human disease. The rat with its fleas has carried bubonic plague from area to area in devastating epidemics since the beginning of history. The body louse, by transmitting typhus, has been responsible for the deaths of more soldiers than all the pre-atomic weapons of mankind. Mosquitoes by transmitting malaria and yellow fever, and tsetse flies by transmitting trypanosomiasis, have depopulated and kept under-populated millions of square miles of fertile land. Even today animal-borne diseases are so widespread and so debilitating, that they profoundly depress agricultural productivity in a world chronically short of food.

The subject is so large that only its more important aspects can be referred to here. We shall be particularly concerned with the control of animal vectors.

MODES OF TRANSMISSION

More than a hundred of the communicable diseases to which man is subject are known to have animal links in their chains of transmission. All the known infective agents are implicated (viruses, rickettsiae, bacteria, fungi, protozoa, and helminths) and the animal vectors include all the common domestic mammals and birds, and many wild vertebrates (mammals, birds and fish), insects and molluscs. In relation to control the way in which the diseases are transmitted is of great importance.

Direct transmission

(*a*) *Physical contact with infected animals.* A number of important infections are acquired by physical contact with infected animals or their carcasses. For example rabies is directly transmitted to man from infected dogs, cats or, in parts of America, vampire bats, and the main source of human anthrax is contact with the carcasses, wool, hair or hides of infected animals or with the feeding stuffs and fertilizers made from the bones and other parts of such animals. Cowpox, rat-bite fever and certain of the dermatomycoses (for example, cat, dog, cattle and horse ringworm) are further examples of diseases directly transmitted by infected animals.

(*b*) *Ingestion of the tissues of infected animals.* Salmonella food poisoning can be transmitted by the ingestion of meat from infected pigs and cows and eggs from infected ducks. In many parts of the world milk from infected animals is responsible for much brucellosis and bovine tuberculosis.

(*c*) *Contact with the excreta of infected animals.* A good example of this type of transmission is provided by Weil's disease. The causal organism (Leptospira icterohaemorrhagica) is excreted in the urine of infected rats and it can survive for several weeks in water, from which it enters the human host through the skin. As a result of this mode of transmission Weil's disease tends to be associated with occupations such as coal mining, sewer work and fish-handling, which bring workers into contact with rat infested waters. Throughout the world salmonellosis is endemic in a wide variety of animals (poultry, swine, cattle and rodents) and food contaminated with the faeces of infected animals can give rise to food poisoning.

Indirect transmission

Much more important are the many infections transmitted indirectly through animal intermediaries or vectors (vertebrate and invertebrate). The modes of transmission are varied and often complex. The vector may act only as a mechanical vehicle for carrying the infecting parasite from one host to another. In this way flies can transfer the organisms of bacillary dysentery from infected faeces to food and cooking utensils—although the usual method of transmission is by direct, person to person contact. More commonly the vector is involved biologically in the process. For example, the rickettsiae of typhus multiply in the cells of the louse midgut and because the louse defaecates as it bites, the human host is inoculated with the infected faeces when he scratches himself. Sometimes the animal vector plays an essential part in the life cycle of the parasite (the sexual cycle of the malaria protozoa takes place only in anopheline mosquitoes). Sometimes several animal intermediaries are involved before a new human host becomes infected: for example the adult fish tapeworm Dyphyllobothrium latum inhabits the human intestine; the eggs are excreted with the faeces, and in fresh water produce free-swimming larvae; the larvae enter the next phase of their development when they are ingested by certain small crustaceans; they undergo further development when the crustaceans are swallowed by small fish; when the small fish are swallowed by larger fish, the larvae invade and become encysted in the muscles of the new hosts; and the cycle is completed when man eats the raw, smoked or pickled flesh of the infected large fish.

The nature of the animal vector (arthropod, mollusc or vertebrate) has an important bearing on the control of indirectly transmitted infections.

(a) Arthropod vectors

Malaria, yellow fever, typhus and trypanosomiasis, all with arthropod vectors, are of the greatest international importance.

(i) Malaria is conveyed only by anopheline mosquitoes. The sporozoites find their way into the insect's salivary glands from which they are injected into the human blood stream when the female mosquito is feeding. The clinical features of the disease are determined by the species of plasmodium involved, and its epidemiological pattern by the habits of fifty or more species of anopheline vectors. All depend upon water for their larval stage, but the choice of water (clean, brackish, tidal, sunlit, shady), flight range, feeding habits and choice of resting place vary from species to species. Climatic conditions are also important; a temperature of not less than 20°C is required before the sexual cycle of P. falciparum (the cause of malignant subtertian malaria) can be completed in the mosquito and a temperature of 15°C is needed for the other species. For this reason it is believed that in historical times malaria was never common in Britain, although indigenous cases still occasionally occur. For example in the years immediately following the First World War 359 cases were notified in Kent, the disease having been transmitted by infected anophelines in the Thames marshes.

(ii) Yellow fever, a virus disease, is also transmitted by mosquitoes. In its epidemic form it is confined to man and is transmitted only by Aedes aegypti, a domestic mosquito which will breed in any small collection of rain water (such as in a discarded tin or motor tyre or the bottom of a boat). The mosquito demands for its life cycle a mean temperature of at least 24°C, so it is confined to the tropics. Although the vector is common in Asia and the Pacific, yellow fever is found only in Africa and South America. In endemic form (jungle yellow fever) the disease occurs sporadically in the scattered rural communities of the tropical rain forests of Africa and South America. This form of the disease has its reservoir in certain species of monkeys and is transmitted from them to man by forest mosquitoes.

(iii) The typhus fevers, due to infection with Rickettsiae, are transmitted by many different arthropods—lice, fleas, ticks and mites. There appears to be no animal reservoir of epidemic typhus, the destroyer of armies and the scourge of hospitals and prisons. It is transmitted from man to man by the body louse, which almost always dies of the infection. All the many other typhus fevers are primarily animal infections, transferred from animal to animal by arthropod vectors and occasionally transmitted to man by the bite of those arthropods. Murine typhus is a world-wide infection of rats, sporadically transmitted to man by infected rat fleas. Dogs and rodents throughout the world are also subject to tick-borne typhus infections, and these are occasionally transmitted to man (as in the examples of Rocky Mounted spotted fever and North Queensland and Kenya typhus).

(iv) Trypanosomiasis, almost confined to Africa, is transmitted by the bite of the tsetse fly, which is biologically involved in the developmental cycle of the protozoa. The different species of the vector are often very specific in their environmental needs, some living only near rivers and streams, others requiring for survival certain shrubs and trees in scrub and bush country. In consequence the human form of the disease, sleeping sickness, is essentially a rural disease, for the vectors cannot survive in an urban environment. Trypanosomiasis of cattle (ngana) is of great medical importance because of its effect upon human nutrition, for it has delayed the development of vast tracts of good grazing land in Central Africa.

(b) Mollusc vectors

Oysters and mussels are sometimes responsible for the spread of typhoid infection, but by far the most important of the mollusc vectors of disease are the freshwater snails which are essential to the life cycle of Schistosoma, the trematode worm responsible for human bilharziasis (the African name for the disease which in other parts of the world is called schistosomiasis). This debilitating disease is widely distributed in Africa, South America, China, Japan and the Philippines. In these countries it is found wherever man comes into barefooted contact with water suitable for the appropriate species of snails. The adult worms live in the human portal system, but the eggs are excreted in the urine and faeces. In water the eggs hatch and the trematode continues its developmental cycle in the tissues of a vector snail, from which it again enters the water to gain access to a human host through the unbroken skin. The disease is very difficult to control and irrigation schemes are introducing it into many fresh areas so that it threatens to replace malaria as the leading vector-borne disease.

(c) Vertebrate vectors

Some of the many worms which parasitize man are transmitted by vertebrate vectors. The human tapeworms Taenia saginata and Taenia solium have cattle and pigs as their intermediate hosts. Gravid segments of the worm are passed in the stools of infected persons and the eggs, if swallowed by the appropriate animal vector, liberate embryos which find their way into the skeletal muscles, where they encyst. Man acquires the worm by eating such muscles raw or incompletely cooked. Man sometimes becomes involved in the life cycle of Echinococcus granulosus. The common definitive host of this small tapeworm is the dog and the usual intermediate host the sheep. Man develops hydatid disease by ingesting the eggs excreted by infected dogs. The disease is an important health problem in many parts of the world and still occurs from time to time in Britain. In a survey of farm dogs in Mid Wales one in five was found to be infected.

CONTROL

It might be expected that of all the major communicable diseases, those in which animals are involved would be most amenable to control, for their epidemiology is well understood, and it should be possible to block the channels of spread by controlling the animal vectors. Yet animal-borne disease remains a major health problem throughout the world. The reasons for this are apparent if we remember what has been achieved in Britain and then consider some of the difficult problems facing less advanced countries.

In Britain the four major animal-borne diseases of historical times have been plague, typhus, bovine tuberculosis and rabies. Plague left the country after the devastating epidemic of 1665, although it remained in parts of Europe for another century. There is no satisfactory explanation for this. Typhus disappeared at the end of the nineteenth century, an unplanned consequence of a rising standard of living (in particular of improved nutrition—the disease in its epidemic form has often accompanied famines) and a decline in the population of body lice associated with changes in clothing habits and patterns of personal cleanliness. In contrast, bovine tuberculosis has been deliberately brought under under control by a programme of public health legislation, aimed first at pasteurization of milk and later at elimination of diseased cattle. Rabies has been eradicated by a combination of chance and choice. The English Channel provides a natural barrier against the entry of infected wild animals and makes it much easier to enforce a rigid quarantine on imported animals.

We are left with a number of less important animal-borne diseases— salmonellosis, brucellosis, leptospirosis, tape-worm infestation and hydatid disease—incompletely controlled by complex statutory machinery concerned with port health, rodent control, refuse disposal, meat inspection and the hygiene of food establishments, slaughter houses and dairies. Control is incomplete because standards of personal hygiene and the cooperation of individuals are also involved.

At a world level the control of the major animal-borne diseases presents formidable problems. The difficulties are well illustrated by the W.H.O. campaign to eliminate malaria, one of the most ambitious health projects of our time. The plan was to achieve global eradication by way of area and regional programmes. The strategy of area eradication is now well defined. It consists of four phases: a preparatory phase usually of about twelve months, in which the malarious area is surveyed and field-workers are trained; an attack phase in which all habitations in the area are sprayed two or three times a year for four years with residual insecticide (at the end of this period almost all malarial infections can be expected to have died out spontaneously); a consolidation phase during which the whole population is kept under surveillance and blood samples are taken from all fever cases in the area, until no new case has been detected for three years; and a maintenance phase to guard against recrudescence or importation of the disease until it has been eradicated in the rest of the world. By these methods malaria has been eradicated in continental Europe, the Mediterranean Islands, the United States and parts of South America, and campaigns are in the consolidation phase in Ceylon and much of India. In many other parts of the world, however, progress is slow. This is partly due to anopheline resistance to insecticides and, in Equatorial Africa, to anopheline vectors that are both unusually efficient and difficult to attack. But the principal cause of incomplete success is breakdown of surveillance during the phase of consolidation through lack of financial and technical resources.

None of the major animal-borne diseases is more difficult to control than bilharziasis. As we have noted, its epidemiology is well understood; yet in most of the affected areas the disease is static and in some, as water resources are developed and irrigation schemes extended, it is spreading. In poor countries with low standards of hygiene it is impossible to prevent the pollution of irrigation water with faeces and urine, and since treatment of the disease is not very effective, agricultural workers inevitably come into contact with infected water.

15 · AIR-BORNE INFECTION

In Britain, respiratory tract infections are the leading cause of general practitioner consultations and absence from work. The common cold is a universal and, so far, an uncontrollable nuisance. Pneumonia, despite effective therapy, remains an important cause of infant mortality and a major cause of death in old age. And in epidemic years morbidity and mortality from influenza are a matter for national concern. When we remember that the specific infections of childhood (chickenpox, whooping cough, measles, mumps, scarlet fever and diphtheria) are also air-borne, it is evident that the control of this method of dissemination of infection is at least as important as the control of water-borne and food-borne disease. It is much more difficult to achieve.

Air had been suspected of playing an important part in the spread of epidemic disease since at least Galen's time. In the second century he wrote 'When many sicken and die at once, we must look to a simple common cause, the air we breathe'. But until Pasteur discredited the notion of spontaneous generation by demonstrating that living organisms can be conveyed through the air, there was no rational basis for the control of airborne infection. The control of water-borne disease preceded the science of bacteriology. Lister's attempt to control airborne surgical sepsis by the use of carbolic acid sprays in operating theatres was derived from it.

Despite the remarkable advances in bacteriological knowledge since Lister's time, control of airborne infection is still far from satisfactory. Technically air is much more difficult to sterilize than water or food. Elimination of organisms from all the air we breathe is quite impossible and is difficult even in the limited environments where there is special need for it (hospital wards and operating theatres). Control of the sources of airborne infection is further complicated by the ubiquity of the common respiratory diseases, by the fact that many of them are infectious before they are clinically apparent (or without ever becoming apparent, as in a subclinical attack or the carrier state), and by the facilities for their spread unavoidably provided in the community (in school, place of work, public transport and public buildings).

MODES OF TRANSMISSION

There are two main methods by which infection is spread through the air: directly from patient to patient by droplets or, more important, droplet nuclei, and indirectly by dust from bedding, clothes, carpets and floors. The methods are not necessarily disease specific. Thus smallpox, pulmonary tuberculosis and streptococcal infections are predominantly transmitted by means of droplet nuclei, they may also be spread by dust. Some of the infections that are normally airborne may be spread by contamination of food, usually milk (for example streptococcal sore throat and diphtheria).

Droplet transmission

During quiet breathing very few droplets are expelled. They are produced by talking, and in much greater numbers by coughing and sneezing. (A sneeze may expel as many as one million droplets.) The largest droplets fall rapidly to the ground or onto the clothes or bedding of the person producing them. Droplets of less than 100 μm in diameter fall more slowly, evaporating as they fall. Depending upon their size, atmospheric humidity, air movement and other factors, a proportion of these smaller droplets lose all their moisture before they reach the ground and remain suspended as droplet nuclei until removed by ventilation. It follows that for infection to be transmitted by droplet spray the susceptible host needs to be very near the source of infection. A child standing close to an infected person is in a particularly vulnerable position. Diseases disseminated mainly by this method are often associated with overcrowded sleeping conditions, as in the case of cerebrospinal meningitis among service personnel, or with close family contact, as in the case of whooping cough. Droplet nuclei, on the other hand, can carry infection over much greater distances. Tubercle bacilli and the viruses of measles, chickenpox and smallpox are commonly disseminated in this way. Because of their small size and low settling velocity the nuclei are readily carried into the alveoli, and it is therefore possible for a susceptible person to become infected from the inhalation of a very small number of them.

Dust transmission

Large droplets, when they fall to the ground, dry out and become part of the dust of the room. If they contain pathogens resistant to drying, the dust may then act as a reservoir of infection for a long time (tubercle bacilli have been known to survive in dust for three months and haemolytic streptococci for six months). Organisms from soiled surgical dressings, skin scales, dried sputum and other secretions can also become part of the dust of a room (cross-infection in surgical wards has often been traced to these sources). However, apart from special places such as hospitals, dust is not a common vehicle for the transmission of air-borne infection. For although huge numbers of particles containing living organisms become air-borne when the dust in a room is disturbed by domestic activities such as sweeping, bed-making and brushing clothes, the great majority of such organisms are not pathogenic.

CONTROL

There are three ways in which control of air-borne infection may be attempted: by removing the source of infection; by interrupting its lines of communication; and by protecting susceptible persons.

Removing the source of infection

In the past the only method which offered any hope of limiting the spread of infection was to isolate from the community those suffering from infectious disease and those who might be incubating an infection because they had been in contact with it. This was the main reason for building fever hospitals in the nineteenth century, although it is doubtful whether they limited the spread of any of the air-borne infections, with the possible exceptions of smallpox and diphtheria. Sanatoria, on the other hand, by isolating for long periods patients with open pulmonary tuberculosis probably contributed to the decline of mortality from the disease during the first half of the present century. Patients with smallpox are still routinely admitted to isolation hospitals. Mortality from the other air-borne infectious diseases (measles, whooping cough, scarlet fever, diphtheria, meningococcal meningitis, influenzal pneumonia, pulmonary tuberculosis) is now so low, and the risk of acquiring a complicating cross-infection in hospital is relatively so much higher, that the crucial reason for hospital admission has become the need for diagnostic and therapeutic facilities rather than for isolation. Indeed, cross-infection is so dangerous to debilitated and susceptible young children that for this reason alone (there are also compelling psychological reasons) sick children should not be admitted to general or paediatric hospitals if they can be treated at home. Sometimes hospital admission is unavoidable, but if there is any suspicion of infection or contact with infection, the child should in the first instance be admitted to an isolation ward.

The classroom, with its crowding together of susceptibles, provides a particularly favourable environment for the transmission of air-borne infection, so children with infectious disease should be kept away from school. The exclusion of contacts, however, although advisable in certain circumstances, no longer needs to be rigorously enforced.

The number of streptococci and staphylococci expelled during ordinary conversation, even from the mouths of known carriers, is small. Nevertheless, the wearing of face masks in operating theatres and delivery rooms remains a sensible precaution. The type of mask is not as important as it was once thought to be, for the organisms are expelled in droplets, not in droplet nuclei, and almost anything placed in front of the mouth will catch them. It is more important that any member of theatre or ward staffs found to be carrying pathogenic organisms in the nasopharynx, for example streptococcus pyogenes or strains of staphalococcus aureus of certain phage types, should be removed from duty.

Interrupting lines of communication

The dissemination of infection by droplets and droplet-nuclei is favoured by confined and crowded working and living conditions. In the open air, infective nuclei are dispersed so rapidly after expulsion that their chance of being inhaled by a susceptible person is negligible. Good ventilation and avoidance of overcrowding are probably still the most effective, as they are certainly the cheapest, methods of reducing the risk of air-borne infection indoors. Florence Nightingale observed that 'if nothing is done for the ventilation, the hospital atmosphere becomes more and more fatal'. In northern latitudes the common respiratory infections and most of the specific fevers of childhood reach their peak incidence during the winter months, when people are crowded indoors, and windows in homes, schools and factories are closed against the weather.

In recognition of the dangers of overcrowding, standards of spacing, usually in terms of floor space per person, are laid down for private houses, and for most public buildings, and Building byelaws require provision of certain facilities for ventilation of domestic and public buildings. The risk of spread of air-borne infection is certainly reduced by ventilation, but experimental work suggests that to eliminate this risk sixty air changes an hour are needed. Ventilation of this kind can be obtained at great cost (usually with much noise) by air-conditioning plant, but it cannot be achieved by ordinary methods without intolerable draughts and insoluble heating problems. For full control of airborne infection, therefore, ventilation needs the support of some method of destroying pathogens in the air.

When used as atomized sprays, sodium hypochlorite, propylene and triethylene glycol, resorcinol, hexylresorcinol and lactic acid have all been shown to sterilize air-borne particles effectively in the laboratory. Field trials, however, have been disappointing, and the only method of aerial disinfection that has so far given encouraging results under field conditions is ultraviolet irradiation. The schoolchild is an important disseminator of respiratory infections, and trials of aerial disinfectants have commonly been focused on air-borne cross-infection in classrooms. When ultraviolet light is used, the upper air of classrooms, cloakrooms and assembly halls is irradiated, and infective droplet nuclei are carried through the bactericidal barrier by the vertical ventilation produced by thermal gradients. In a large scale trial by the Air Hygiene Committee of the Medical Research Council, three primary schools in Southall, London, were equipped with ultravoilet lamps and three comparable schools in the same area were used as controls. Over a three year period irradiation produced a substantial reduction in airborne Streptococcus salivarius, and a less marked reduction in the incidence of measles, chickenpox and mumps. But there was little or no difference between irradiated schools and controls in the incidence of coryza, febrile catarrh and other common respiratory infections. The results suggest that irradiation of the upper air of large rooms checks the spread of infections disseminated by droplet nuclei but, as might be expected, is much less effective against the infections disseminated by droplet spray and the contamination of hands, clothes, handkerchiefs and floor dust.

Control of dust-borne infection is of great importance in hospitals. Floor-sweeping and bed-making disturb myriads of dust particles, and staphylococci and haemolytic streptococci can readily be recovered from the floors and bedding of surgical wards. During the Second World War, cross-infection in military hospitals was not uncommonly traced to this source, and the emergence of antibiotic-resistant pathogens has heightened the need for control. Oil treatment of floors and bedding reduces very substantially the amount of dust in wards and the use of vacuum cleaners with appropriate filters is even more effective. At points of high risk (such as operating theatres, burns units and labour wards) dust can be removed from the incoming air by filtration or electro-static precipitation, the air sterilized by ultraviolet irradiation, and the dispersal of infective particles checked by introducing clean air from above and removing it at floor level. It must be remembered, however, that these protective measures do not eliminate the risk of cross-infection from droplet spray or direct contact, methods of spread favoured by resistant strains of staphylococcus aureus. Human reservoirs of infection must also be identified and treated.

Protecting susceptible populations

It is so difficult to block all the channels by which air-borne infection can be transmitted that for the common respiratory infections prophylactic immunization appears to offer the only hope of full control. By this means diphtheria has already been virtually banished from Britain. B.C.G. is making a substantial contribution towards the eradication of tuberculosis, and an effective vaccine has greatly reduced mortality from whooping cough. Trials of measles vaccines are promising, and gamma-globulin can be used to prevent or modify the disease in very young or sick and debilitated older children. Progress towards the control of influenza is slow. Virus-specific vaccines provide reasonable protection, but vaccines are of limited value when the epidemic virus has a different antigenic pattern from the viruses in the vaccine. Whisky remains one of the pleasantest of the many ineffective prophylactics against the common cold.

16 · ATMOSPHERIC POLLUTION

This chapter is concerned with the causes, effects on health and control of pollution of urban atmosphere from domestic and industrial sources. The relation between tobacco smoke and ill-health is discussed in Chapter 10 and the effects and control of atmospheric pollution at place of work in Chapter 18.

In towns both clean air and safe water depend on the control of domestic and industrial effluents; but whereas the problem of controlling the pollution of water supplies was well on the way to being solved by the end of the nineteenth century (the first and most notable success of the public health movement) the problem of controlling urban atmospheric pollution is still with us. This is partly because pollution of the air is more difficult and costly to control, and partly because its connection with ill-health is more complex and not so easily demonstrated. In Britain the cholera epidemics of the middle of the nineteenth century provided alarming and unmistakable evidence of the need to separate sewage from drinking water. It was not until a century later that the London smog disaster of 1952 gave an equally dramatic demonstration of the need to control atmospheric pollution.

CAUSES AND COMPOSITION OF POLLUTION

The main sources of atmospheric pollution are the domestic and industrial combustion of solid fuel (coal and coke) and of petroleum products (kerosene, diesel oil and motor spirit). In Britain at the present time only about one sixth of the solid fuel and one twentieth of the oil consumed is used in homes; the rest goes to industry and to road and rail transport.

The solid components of pollution may be classified as grit, dust and smoke. Grit consists of gross particles upwards of 76 μm in diameter, dust of smaller particles down to 1 μm, and smoke of particles of less than 1 μm. Nearly all the grit and dust discharged into the air comes from industrial sources. (In domestic fireplaces the large particles remain behind in the grate as ash, but in industrial furnaces they are driven up the chimneys by the much higher temperatures.) Because of its weight, grit tends to settle in the immediate neighbourhood of industrial chimneys, but dust particles are dispersed more widely. On the other hand nearly all the smoke pollution comes from incomplete combustion of coal. (Oil and coke fuels make a very small contribution.) Although only about one-sixth of the national consumption of coal is used for domestic purposes, half of the low-level smoke in industrial districts comes from domestic grates which burn raw coal very inefficiently. In industry, coal is used more efficiently, and the combustion products are usually discharged into the upper air from tall chimney stacks. There is an appreciable quantity of benzpyrene in coal smoke and minute but measurable amounts of that known carcinogen are present in the atmospheres of our towns and cities.

The combustion of coal and oil produces a wide range of gaseous pollutants. From British coal over five million tons of sulphur dioxide are discharged into the air every year. In large industrial towns the mean atmospheric concentration of sulphur dioxide during the winter months is about 0·2 parts per million, and in smog episodes it has risen to over one part per million. The nitrogen oxides emitted from the chimneys of industrial furnaces and exhausts of internal combustion engines may also be of pathological significance. They are present as a regular pollutant in the air of the cities of Britain at concentrations of about 0·1 parts per million. There is very little carbon monoxide in flue gas, but it constitutes 10 per cent of the exhaust gas from internal combustion engines. Concentrations of two parts per million are common in traffic congested city streets, and may reach thirty or more times that level in traffic tunnels or in traffic jams. Fuel burning produces huge quantities of carbon dioxide (it is poured into the atmosphere at a rate of over 200 million tons a year) but it is diluted so rapidly that it does not constitute a toxic hazard.

The concentration of pollutants in the atmosphere of a town is determined in the first place by the quantities discharged into the air from local industrial and domestic sources. An important secondary influence is the rate at which pollutants are subsequently removed from the air. Particles of grit and dust settle by gravitation. The rate at which smoke and gases are dispersed depends upon rainfall, the direction and force of prevailing winds, and upon air turbulence created by geographical contours and thermal gradients. The sun warms the earth and this sets up convection currents by warming the air at its surface. The warm air rises, carrying with it and dispersing the pollutants. Under anti-cyclonic weather conditions, usually aided by a local topography which restricts air flow, a temperature inversion may occur with the warm air above and the cold air below. When this happens there is no upward movement of air, and in a heavily polluted area pollutants can accumulate to produce a 'smog episode', with immediate effects on the health of the local population (see below).

EFFECTS UPON HEALTH

For a number of reasons the effect of atmospheric pollution on health is difficult to measure. In the first place the acute effects are nonspecific; smog episodes produce an increase in morbidity and mortality among those already suffering from cardiac or pulmonary disability rather than a specific and clearly recognizable illness. Second, the long-term effects can be estimated only by their contribution to the complex, multifactorial aetiology of chronic bronchitis and cancer of the lung. Third, atmospheric pollution has many different components, particulate and gaseous, and their effects are unusually difficult to separate. Even in the controlled environment of the animal laboratory the effects of pollution are difficult to separate and to measure. It has been shown, however, that when mice are exposed to quite low concentrations of sulphur dioxide their growth is stunted and they develop recognizable pathological changes in the lungs. It is also known that skin and lung cancers can be produced by exposing them to the polycyclic hydrocarbons found in the atmosphere of cities.

Immediate effects

The immediately harmful effect of gross atmospheric pollution has been impressively demonstrated by three major smog episodes: in

December 1930, in the Meuse Valley, Belgium; in October 1948, in the city of Donora, United States; and in December 1952, in London. All three episodes were characterized by anticyclonic weather conditions, high atmosphere humidity (producing fog), and an unusually persistent thermal inversion which allowed pollutants to accumulate in the still air for several days. In London all the pollutants were products of coal combustion, but in the Meuse Valley and in Donora some of them came from heavy industry (coke ovens, blast furnaces, zinc reduction plant, etc.).

In the London episode the pollutants began to accumulate on December 5th and reached their maximum concentration within three days. The amount of sulphur dioxide in the air increased seven times and the concentration of suspended matter (smoke) ten times; but it was only after retrospective analysis of mortality and morbidity data that the gravity of the episode was appreciated. In the smog area there was an excess of 1,600 deaths during the first three weeks of December, mainly among infants and the elderly. Table 22 shows that much of

Table 22. Deaths registered in London Administrative County for the smog episode of 1952

Cause of death	Number of deaths		
	(a) Week of Smog	(b) Week before Smog	Ratio a/b
Bronchitis	704	74	9·3
Respiratory tuberculosis	77	14	5·5
Influenza and pneumonia	192	47	4·1
Other respiratory diseases	52	9	4·8
Coronary disease and myocardial degeneration	525	206	2·6
All other conditions	934	595	1·6
Total	2,484	945	2·6

the excess was due to a very large rise in mortality from all the major respiratory diseases; but the number of deaths attributed to coronary disease and myocardial degeneration also increased substantially. From hospital admissions, sickness claims and general practitioners' records there is evidence that although the amount of respiratory illness in the population increased steeply, the increase was less than might have been expected from the number of deaths. The general conclusion drawn from the evidence was that the main effect of the smog was to exacerbate illness and precipitate death among people with pre-existing respiratory or cardiac conditions.

The eye and lung irritating photochemical smogs of Los Angeles are produced by an interaction of ozone and the hydrocarbons and oxides of nitrogen from the exhausts of motor vehicles in the still air and bright sunlight of that city. In Britain the necessary concentration of motor vehicles exists in some of the large cities, but there is not enough still air and bright sunlight to cause this unpleasant phenomenon.

Long-term effects

There is much evidence to suggest that in industrialized communities atmospheric pollution plays some part in the aetiology of chronic bronchitis and carcinoma of the lung. It is difficult to assess the precise part, however, for the evidence is indirect (most of it derived from epidemiological studies in Britain) and difficult to interpret.

To begin with, the excessively high death rate from chronic bronchitis in the United Kingdom is often attributed to enthusiasm for coal fires. But bronchitis is a notoriously imprecise diagnosis, and some of the excess is undoubtedly due to the national tendency to give bronchitis as the cause of death. There are also considerable differences between countries in smoking habits, and tobacco is a very important aetiological influence (Chapter 10). Then there is the relation between size of town and mortality from bronchitis and cancer of the lung, referred to in Chapter 5. This may be due in part to the higher concentration of pollutants in larger towns; but other features of urban life may also be important, for example overcrowding (which increases the risk of recurrent respiratory infection), and the gross atmospheric pollution to which some men are exposed at their place of work.

The case against atmospheric pollution as the cause of part of the increase of bronchitis and lung cancer mortality with increasing population density is strengthened by the observation that mortality from bronchitis in the county boroughs is directly related to intensity of air pollution. Even more convincing are the results of a survey of sickness absence, premature retirement and death among postmen, in which indices of population density, household crowding and atmospheric pollution were defined and morbidity and mortality rates calculated by cause for different areas. Disablement and death from bronchitis were found to be closely related to urban pollution but not to area or domestic crowding. In contrast, mortality from carcinoma of the lung was much more closely related to population density; and morbidity from influenza was related to household overcrowding.

The rapidly increasing density of the traffic on the roads raises questions about the possible effects on health of the carbon monoxide and lead expelled at street level from motor exhausts into the air of our towns. The levels of carboxyhaemoglobin registered in the bloods of people exposed to atmospheric pollution from heavy traffic are regularly exceeded by the levels found in the blood of cigarette smokers not exposed to traffic pollution, but it must be remembered that the two effects can be additive. So far the blood lead levels recorded in people exposed to motor exhaust fumes in cities, although some cause for concern, have been well below the levels at which overt lead intoxication occurs.

In conclusion, there is little doubt that long-term exposure to atmospheric pollution contributes to the high prevalence of bronchitis and lung cancer in Britain, although the effect is difficult to quantify. It is also likely that by increasing the general gloom and squalor of industrialized cities it makes a contribution to mental ill-health, and by screening the sunlight it may stunt the growth of city children.

CONTROL

In Britain awareness of the smoke nuisance and the need for its control has a long history. In 1273 the burning of coal in London was prohibited by statute and in 1306 an artificer was executed for the offence. Queen Elizabeth I was 'greatly grieved and annoyed with the taste and smoke of the sea-coals'. In 'Fumifugium: or the smoke of London Dissipated', John Evelyn in 1661 submitted to Charles II a plan to control the 'hellish and dismal cloud' which enveloped London. And since the middle of the nineteenth century there has been an accumulation of statutory attempts to control pollution from industrial sources. Yet, after seven centuries of endeavour, atmospheric pollution remains a major problem in the field of environmental hygiene. The reasons are not far to seek. For centuries coal has been the cheapest and most accessible source of power for industry and of heat for the home. Growth of population and industrial expansion have continued to outpace unpopular attempts to control pollution, unpopular because they tend to increase the cost of industrial processes, and because the open-hearth fire is a long established feature of domestic architecture and winters are not quite cold enough to force a break with tradition. Before reviewing the present position, we will mention briefly some of the problems of control.

Cleaning the air of cities requires control of emission of pollutants from the burning of fuel for domestic and industrial purposes. There is little prospect of developing domestic apparatus for burning raw coal without smoke, and the solution to the domestic problem is the use of gas, electricity and oil or of solid smokeless fuels (such as coke, anthracite, coalite and phurnacite) in properly designed appliances, supplemented possibly by district heating schemes. Control of emission of pollutants from conventional power stations and from industrial processes is more complex. If appropriate methods are used, almost any fuel can be burnt without the emission of dust or smoke. But control of harmful waste gases, particularly sulphur dioxide, is more difficult. The long-term solution to the sulphur dioxide problem lies in increasing use of sulphur-free fuels and of atomic and hydroelectric sources of power. In the meantime aesthetic considerations are put aside and we rely upon rapid dilution of irritant flue gases to safe levels by discharging them into the upper air through tall, unsightly chimneys.

For the first half of the twentieth century, legislation to control atmospheric pollution was fragmentary, permissive and never very effective. The London smog of 1952 disclosed the urgency and magnitude of the problem. The following year the Government appointed a Committee 'to examine the nature, causes and effects of air pollution and the efficiency of present preventive measures; to consider what further preventive measures are practicable; and to make recommendations'. The Committee reported in 1954 and the Clean Air Acts of 1956 and 1968 embodied most of the recommendations. Emission of black smoke from chimneys is prohibited; new industrial furnaces may not be installed unless they are provided with grit arresting equipment and are capable, so far as practicable, of being operated without emitting smoke; and local authorities are empowered to declare 'smoke control areas' in which the emission of smoke from chimneys is an offence. Since the Acts the amount of smoke discharged into the atmosphere from industrial sources has been uniformly reduced. The effect upon domestic sources of pollution has been much less uniform. London and a few large cities have substantially lowered the levels of atmospheric pollution with a noticeable effect upon age standardized death rates from bronchitis. Other cities and towns have been less enthusiastic in use of the power given to them under the Acts.

FURTHER READING

Report of the Royal College of Physicians (1970) *Air Pollution and Health*. Pitman Medical and Scientific Publishing Co. Ltd., London.
Reports on Public Health and Medical Reports (1954) *Mortality and Morbidity during the London Fog of December 1952*. H.M.S.O.

17 · THE HOME

The association between ill-health and adverse living conditions, although more immediately obvious than that between disease and dirty food or water, is also more complex. People who live in unsatisfactory houses are usually poor, and it is difficult to separate the effect of bad housing from the many other adverse environmental influences associated with poverty. To this must be added the complication of the question posed by Karl Pearson: how much of the high mortality in slum areas is due to bad housing and how much to 'the drifting of physically and mentally inferior sections of the people into these dwellings by a process of selection'.

There are three principal ways in which housing may affect health: first, through the structure of the house (a matter of bricks, mortar and equipment); second, through the relation between size of the house and the number of people living in it (a matter of overcrowding); and third, through the situation of the house (a matter of neighbourhood conditions and amenities). Although these unhealthy influences are commonly found together, presenting the problem of overcrowding in substandard houses packed closely together in an unfavourable environment and without social amenities, it will be convenient to consider them separately.

Substandard houses

Badly built, dilapidated and poorly equipped houses are the direct cause of much ill-health. Without an indoor hot-water supply, dirt and refuse accumulate, vermin are encouraged and the spread of infection is facilitated. When cooking facilities are inadequate and the larder is an unventilated cupboard under the stairs, there is likely to be wasteful buying, an ill-balanced diet and an increased risk of food-borne infection. Uneven floors, steep stairs without handrails, bad lighting and dilapidated furniture and household fittings, lead to accidents in the home, particularly in young children and old people.

Overcrowding

It is easy to understand why overcrowding also causes much ill-health. When large families are living together in one room during the day-time and sleeping several to a bedroom, opportunities for the spread of air-borne infection are greatly increased. Young children are particularly vulnerable. Infections are brought into the home by older brothers and sisters, and the earlier in infancy the common infections are acquired the more likely they are to prove fatal or to result in chronic ill-health.

Overcrowding may also have harmful psychological effects. When people are living too close together, irritability and frustration due to clashes of temperament and interests are inevitable; lack of privacy makes it impossible to hide these conflicts from children. Over-crowding in the bedroom—children with parents, older children with younger children, brothers with sisters—may lead to emotionally disturbing sexual experiences. The schoolchild has no space for play or for study, and the adolescent is not encouraged to bring friends into the home. The wheel comes full circle when young couples cannot find a house of their own and are forced to spend the formative years of their married lives in the overcrowded houses in which they were born.

Neighbourhood amenities

The ill effects of living in substandard houses are often augmented by a lack of social and recreational amenities in the neighbourhood. It would be surprising if poor quality houses crowded together in a district short of school accommodation and health centres and devoid of clubs and playing fields did not have an adverse effect on the physical and mental health of those living in them. Two obvious consequences are that adolescents have nowhere to meet except at street corners and children have nowhere to play except on the streets or in derelict houses. The problem of the effect on health of lack of social amenities is not limited to pockets of bad housing in the older parts of our industrial towns. Many of the housing estates built between the wars were designed without a full appreciation of the need for such amenities.

PUBLIC CONTROL OF HOUSING

When we speak of housing as a social problem we are referring to working-class housing, and the crux of that problem has always been how to provide accommodation at rentals that the average wage earner can afford. The cost of satisfactory housing, like the cost of education and of medical care, puts it beyond the unaided reach of large sections of the population. The rapid increase in population has made it difficult to build enough houses to keep pace with needs; it has also hampered state control of standards and delayed demolition of inadequate old property.

When the population was small and mainly rural there were no great aggregations of slum property and the bad living conditions of the poor presented no obvious threat to the health of the well-to-do. But from the middle of the eighteenth century, with the rapid growth of population due to the Industrial Revolution, the situation began to change. Rural labourers poured into the rapidly expanding industrial towns, and squalid clusters of back-to-back, terrace and courtyard houses, without water or sanitation, were thrown up by speculative builders to accommodate them. These houses were probably no worse than the rural hovels the labourers had come from—indeed they may even have been better. But there were far more of them and they were packed more closely together. By the middle of the nineteenth century the evil consequences were obvious to the eye and nose; and the recurrent threat of cholera led to Government action. The Artisans' and Labourers' Dwellings Act (1868) authorized local authorities to repair, or, if necessary, to demolish without compensation, houses 'unfit for human habitation'. This was followed before the end of the century by legislation which empowered them to condemn, demolish and reconstruct whole areas. But, although some of the larger cities (notably Birmingham and Manchester) made good use of their powers to enforce repair of dilapidated houses and to demolish slum property, few new houses were built by local authorities.

Nevertheless, some progress was made. For census purposes overcrowding has been measured as the proportion of persons (children counted as half and infants not counted) living at more than two per room in households of less than five rooms. (By modern standards this is a very inadequate index: a family consisting of a man, his wife and six children living in a three-roomed tenement would not be classed as overcrowded.) In 1891 the percentage of overcrowding in the population was 7·9; by 1911 it had fallen to 5·1. Between 1914 and 1918 building was at a standstill and after the war there was an acute shortage of working-class accommodation. The need was urgent. Objections to subsidized public enterprise were ignored, and substantial exchequer grants were made available for municipal schemes. Although the amount of subsidy and the method by which it has been paid has since varied greatly, the policy of providing financial help from central funds for the building of working-class houses has remained. Of the four million houses built between the wars, one-and-a-half million were State aided. Since the war considerably more than half the new houses have been built by local authorities, and at the 1951 census only 1·1 per cent of the population was still 'over-crowded'.

State subsidies have had two important results: they have increased the rate at which working-class houses are built; and they have substantially raised the standard of these houses. At the beginning of the present century a shared outdoor lavatory was the rule, an indoor water supply was uncommon and a bathroom was unheard of. Today new houses must conform with specified standards of room size, living space and natural lighting; and they must be equipped with satisfactory cooker, sink and larder, and with adequate washing and storage facilities as well as hot and cold water, indoor sanitation and a bathroom. Yet a very substantial proportion of houses is still seriously inadequate. Local authorities have wide powers to inspect in their areas and may order the repair of dilapidated houses and the demolition of those 'unfit for human habitation'. But the cessation of all building and destruction of many houses during the war, immigration since the war and the still increasing population have seriously hampered the application of these powers.

It is now generally recognized that there must be both public subsidy and public control of standards if the majority of families are to be reasonably housed. There must also be control of the siting of houses and the planning of the neighbourhood in which they are built. Town planning is not a new idea. In the early nineteenth century Napoleon did for Paris what Wren in the seventeenth century had hoped to do for London; and the terraces, squares and crescents of Regents Park, Bath and Cheltenham provide good examples of effective planning in the eighteenth century. But these are isolated examples and public control at the national level is a recent innovation and has been taken seriously only since the Town and Country Planning Act, 1947.

HOUSING AND HEALTH

That there is a close association between poor living conditions and ill-health has been generally accepted and has provided ammunition for social reformers for more than a hundred years. It has also led to vigorous public action. Yet there is little numerical evidence of the precise part played by the various elements of bad housing in the aetiology of disease, disability and death. It is interesting to compare this situation with the general attitude towards evidence connecting tobacco with cancer of the lung and chronic bronchitis. Here the evidence of a close association is statistically unassailable, but as yet little public action has been taken.

It is easy to demonstrate that people who live in districts where the housing is bad are less healthy than those who live in areas where it is good. At corresponding ages their children are shorter and more likely to suffer from skin infections, to have defective vision and hearing, and to die from pneumonia, enteritis and the common infections of childhood. In adult life they have a higher mortality from tuberculosis, rheumatic heart disease, chronic bronchitis and many other diseases. However, evidence of this type (and there is much of it) does not prove that bad housing is itself directly responsible for high mortality. The worst houses are closest together and most overcrowded, and are occupied by the poorest and largest families. The diet of such families is sometimes deficient in quantity and often badly balanced; the wage earners in poor families have the lowest standard of medical care. In effect high mortality rates in slum areas provide evidence, not so much of a relation between ill-health and bad housing, as of a relation between ill-health and poverty, of which a poor standard of housing is an obvious attribute.

Except in respect of accidents in the home, there is probably no clear evidence that substandard housing of itself can affect health directly. It is widely held that cold, damp and insanitary living conditions play a part in promoting chronic and acute rheumatic disease.

Acute rheumatism was made notifiable in Sheffield in 1947. Between 1948 and 1950 it was three times more common among unskilled workers than among the professional and admistrative classes. But there was little difference between patients and controls in respect of standard of housing (structure, ventilation, light, damp, cleanliness, etc.). However, the risk was found to be greater in large than in small families and in schoolchildren than in pre-school children.

The evidence connecting overcrowding and ill-health is rather more convincing, although it is not easy to separate this aspect of the domestic environment from the under-nutrition, and lack of sanitary, washing and cooking facilities often associated with it.

The risk of children contracting lower respiratory infections during the first two years of life has been shown to be greater in overcrowded homes, particularly when bedrooms were shared with parents or other children. Children in overcrowded homes also catch measles and whooping cough earlier and are more likely to die from those diseases.

The relation between respiratory tuberculosis and overcrowding might be expected to be clear cut. It is not. There is no difficulty in demonstrating that overcrowded areas of large towns have higher notification rates and mortality than less crowded areas; but the relationship is not so obvious in the households of patients. This is not to deny the importance of household contact with an open case in the spread of disease; but the effect of overcrowding *per se* appears to be less important than one might expect.

In conclusion it has to be admitted that the evidence connecting bad housing and overcrowding with disease is unsatisfactory. But even if it were possible to apportion the precise contribution of insanitary housing and overcrowding to morbidity and mortality from infectious disease and accident, this would probably represent only a small part of the damage done to the mental and physical health of the community by bad living conditions. The improvement in home conditions in the first half of the twentieth century has undoubtedly played a part in lowering national mortality and improving national health.

SOME PRESENT DAY PROBLEMS

In 1949 the Royal Commission on Population recommended that one person per room should be the maximum permitted density for any household. In 1971 nearly two million people in Great Britain were still living at a mean density of over one and a half persons per room. In addition, 18 per cent of households were still without an inside water closet, 15 per cent without a fixed bath and 12 per cent without a hot water tap. This shortage of accommodation and of household amenities raises the problem of priorities among families on the waiting list as new houses become available. Justice must appear to be done, and most local authorities have points schemes which take account of family size, degree of overcrowding, ill-health, state of existing accommodation, war service, length of residence in the area, etc. Health reasons for priority are also recognized: for example the need for a separate bedroom for a member of the family who has respiratory tuberculosis; and ground floor accommodation for a person suffering from advanced cardiac disease or crippling arthritis.

Some families seem incapable of managing the machinery of ordinary family life or of using effectively the health and welfare services available to them. In these families poverty is not so much the cause of trouble as one of its symptoms. Perhaps the most characteristic feature of such problem families is the squalor of their home life, which leads to ill-health and premature death of children. From the landlord's point of view they are unsatisfactory tenants and tend to drift into the meanest quarters of the slums; and if rehoused in a new housing estate, they soon turn their new homes into slums. Surveys since the war suggest that about one family in 200 is of this type. Some are social casualties (their bad living conditions are due to chronic ill-health or death of husband or wife), and with financial help and a little guidance they can be rehabilitated. Most, however, can only be called social defectives; one or both parents is not uncommonly mentally handicapped. Some problem families can be helped a little by substantial outside support and guidance of the type provided by the social services departments of local authorities and voluntary welfare associations; but in spite of social assistance others deteriorate. The ultimate sanction against such families is to remove the children from their parents as 'being in need of care and protection'. But the break-up or segregation of the problem family can never be more than an administrative expedient.

In large cities the rehousing of people from slum clearance areas presents many problems. The choice lies between blocks of flats in the clearance areas, which are usually near the city centre (these have a great attraction for architect and town planner but are much less attractive to the mother with a young family), new estates near the city's edge (which extend the suburban sprawl), or new satellite towns (a long-term policy with its own peculiar difficulties). Wherever the site, the need is not only for new houses, but for a new community with a social life of its own. The provision of shopping and community centres, schools and health centres, playing fields, open spaces, public houses and churches should be as much part of a rehousing scheme as the provision of bathrooms, adequate bedroom space and good facilities for preparing, cooking and storing food. A balanced community should take into account the needs of the young and the old, and of small families and large. It should also make provision for growth and change.

Other current difficulties include: the special and still largely unmet needs of the increasing number of old people; the extent to which housing shortages hamper the redeployment of labour, so necessary to the national economy when many old industries are dying and new ones being developed; the inadequate provision for large families at one end of the scale and for single people seeking separate accommodation at the other; the special needs of the homeless; and above all the growing problem of housing coloured people.

18 · PLACE OF WORK

In Britain twentyfive million men and women spend half their waking hours at paid work outside their homes. The jobs they do are extremely varied and expose them to a bewildering range of environments. Some workplaces are old, badly lighted, poorly ventilated, inadequately heated, and short of even the basic amenities; others have high standards of hygiene and house-keeping and provide excellent health and welfare services. Some occupations make heavy physical demands while others are sedentary; some are associated with well-recognized hazards (lead, mercury, carbon monoxide, ionizing radiations) and many others carry less clearly defined risks of ill-health and accidents; a few are intellectually and emotionally satisfying, but most are tedious and unrewarding.

Clearly, the working environment must have a considerable influence on health. The subject is extensive. There are many textbooks, scientific papers and government publications on occupational hygiene, industrial toxicology, industrial psychology, industrial diseases and occupational health services. Even to summarize the wide range of problems involved would be outside the scope of this book and we must limit ourselves to a brief discussion of some of the more important aspects of the subject. First we shall look at the structure of the working population. Next we shall consider the ways in which the working environment may affect health. Then we shall indicate the methods by which adverse influences in that environment may be controlled. Finally we shall review the position of occupational health services in the country.

THE WORKING POPULATION

In 1971 the population of Great Britain was 54 millions. Table 23 shows the distribution of the 25 million men and women in gainful employment by types of employment and types of industries and services. More than one third of them (38·2 per cent) were working in the manufacturing industries upon which the prosperity of the country mainly depends (engineering and electrical goods, metal

Table 23. Distribution of the working population of Great Britain, June 1971

Employment Structure	Millions	Percentage
Employees in employment	22·0	88·7
Employers and self-employed	1·7	6·9
H.M. Forces and women's services	0·4	1·6
Wholly unemployed	0·7	2·8
Total working population	24·8	100%
Distribution of employees by industry		
Agriculture, forestry, fishing, mining, quarrying	0·7	3·2
Manufacturing	8·4	38·2
Construction	1·2	5·5
Public utilities (gas, electricity, water)	0·4	1·8
Transport and communication	1·6	7·3
Distributive trades	2·6	11·8
Financial, professional, scientific and other services (including catering)	5·7	25·9
Public administration	1·4	6·4
Total employees in employment	22·0	100%

manufacture, vehicles, textiles, leather, clothing and footwear, chemicals and allied industries, food, drink and tobacco, etc.) one quarter (25·9 per cent) were providing financial, professional, scientific and other services (including hotels and catering), and only 3·2 per cent were working in the basic industries of agriculture, forestry, fishing, mining and quarrying.

One of the more striking changes in the structure of the working population in recent years has been the increase in the proportion of married women in employment: 42 per cent of all married women are at work and women now make up more than one third of the total working population. Another important feature of industrialization in Britain is the large number of small factories. More than half of the persons in gainful employment work in factories employing 250 or fewer persons; about a million of them are in factories employing twentyfive or fewer persons. This adds greatly to the difficulty of ensuring safe and healthy working conditions for all industrial workers.

WORK AND HEALTH

Here we consider briefly the many ways in which health may be adversely affected by the working environment. Harmful influences sometimes make their presence obvious in a dramatic and unmistakable manner by causing acute illness or sudden death (as in cyanide poisoning and electric shock) or by giving rise to conditions long recognized as having an occupational aetiology (such as silicosis and mercurialism). Sometimes the influence, although direct and specific, is less obvious because of the long latent period between exposure and development of symptoms (as in the production of bladder cancer by β-naphthylamine and mesothelioma by asbestos). Sometimes the influence of the working environment is difficult to separate from other known or suspected factors in the aetiology of a disease (for example chronic bronchitis in coal miners). There is also the effect—subtle, indirect and difficult to measure—of poor working conditions upon morale, efficiency, sickness absence and accident rates.

The physical environment

(a) Heat

In some occupations workers are exposed to extremes of heat, or less commonly, of cold, and unless properly protected may become acutely ill. For example, stokers, foundry workers, miners and others doing heavy work at high temperatures may develop 'heat cramps' due to excessive sweating; workers exposed to the low temperatures of refrigerated stores are liable to chilblains, and if inadequately protected, may develop frost-bite or even gangrene. Exposure to such extremes of temperature is uncommon, and when unavoidable the need for protective measures is obvious. But conditions of thermal discomfort far short of the extremes have been shown to lower the quantity and quality of work done, and to increase accident rates, absenteeism and labour turnover. The sensation of being uncomfortably hot or cold is complex. The radiant temperature of the solid surroundings, the temperature and humidity of the ambient air, ventilation (air move-ment), physical activity and the type of clothing worn all play their part. Under ordinary conditions air temperatures within the range 15–22°C are considered comfortable by most people doing light or sedentary work. But what is a comfortable temperature for one person may cause discomfort for another, and standards of comfort vary greatly from country to country. In most American hotels air tempera-tures are above the upper end of the range; in many English hotels they are at the lower end and sometimes below it. In industry the question of thermal comfort is complicated by the fact that some occupations are unavoidably associated with high, low or fluctuating temperatures, high humidity or excessive air movement. Summarizing indices have been devised and comfort zones mapped out; but in most places thermal comfort is still assured by rule of thumb adjust-ment after complaint, so that uncomfortable working temperatures are probably the cause of much industrial inefficiency.

(b) Light

The effects that inadequate lighting, shadows, flicker, glare and too much contrast have upon fatigue, eyestrain and liability to accidents are well known and are supported by convincing evidence from laboratory experiment and from observations in industry. The need for a good light at working level is generally appreciated, and the intensity and quality of illumination are readily measured by the photometer and daylight meter. Several occupations with unusual light conditions carry special health hazards. Many miners who had worked for years at the coal face by the light of flame safety lamps (introduced because of the methane fire risk) developed miner's nystagmus, with its overlay of psychoneurotic symptoms. This troublesome and once common condition has disappeared with the improved lighting at the coal face. Acute and painful oedema of the cornea ('arc eye') can appear abruptly one or two hours after even a momentary exposure to the intense ultra-violet radiation emitted by arc and gas welding apparatus.

(c) Noise

Engineers are making town and factory life noisier, and there are serious grounds for concern about the effect on health and working efficiency. In the nineteenth century it was known that noisy occupations (boiler-making, rivetting, cotton weaving) could cause deafness. Refined methods developed in recent years for measuring auditory acuity and intensity of noise and its component frequencies have increased awareness of the effects of a noisy working environment. Intensity, pitch and regularity of noise and duration of exposure all need to be taken into account. In general, auditory acuity at the higher frequencies is affected first. Impairment at 4,000 Hertz and above can often be detected long before a worker himself is conscious of any hearing loss. However, when the impairment extends downwards into the speech range (below 2,000 Hz) it becomes an obvious social handicap. A given intensity of noise is more damaging if it is concentrated in a narrow band at the higher frequencies than if spread across the frequency range. It is now recognized that the threshold level of noise above which hearing damage can be caused is 85–90 dBA (decibels with an 'A' weighting on the sound meter) and the Department of Employment recommends that for an eight hour working day 90 dBA should not be exceeded. The higher the level the greater the risk of damage and the shorter the exposure needed to cause it—a few minutes exposure to levels above 135 dBA can cause severe and irreversible damage to the organ of Corti. Some observations in industry suggest that levels below 90 dBA, although very unlikely to damage hearing, may cause an irritability and fatigue which leads to a lowered output and an increased accident risk.

(d) Other influences

At place of work, as at home and elsewhere, crowding and poor ventilation facilitate the spread of airborne infection (Chapter 15). There is some evidence that in relation to the spread of pulmonary tuberculosis and upper respiratory infections the number of workers in a workroom or an office is more important than the amount of floor space per worker (because the greater the number of possible contacts the greater the risk). Finally we should mention that poor hygiene in a works canteen may cause an outbreak of food poisoning and in dirty occupations lack of proper washing facilities increases the risk of dermatitis.

The psychological environment

Inimical physical environments may produce serious disease such as stoker's cramp, miner's nystagmus and boilermaker's deafness. Today these conditions do not often occur, and when they do the danger to health is so obvious that the worker is almost always protected. Lesser deviations from physical comfort, however, are still common. Their effect is largely psychological and can be measured only indirectly. We have already mentioned that thermal discomfort, poor lighting and excessive noise appear to influence productivity, absenteeism, accident rates and labour turnover. However, the well-known experiments carried out by Elton Mayo at the Hawthorn works of the Western Electric Company in Chicago between 1924 and 1927 indicated that the relationship between physical conditions at work and psychological well-being is not as straightforward as had previously been thought. A series of improvements in working conditions of a group of workers led to considerable increases in output; but output remained high when all improvements were withdrawn. Mayo concluded, plausibly if somewhat obviously, that people work better if someone in authority takes an interest in them: job satisfaction is important. Bad working conditions may cause psychoneurotic disturbances; but bad working conditions are often a sign of lack of interest by management and of unsatisfactory relationships within the working group.

Psychological techniques developed in the laboratory are now applied fairly widely in personnel selection and are also used in the study of working practices and design of machines and equipment. They are not yet much applied to the problem of communications in industry (or medicine). People like to know what is going on but often they are not told. Firm decisions based on adequate consultation and communicated clearly are good for morale; incompletely understood rules and contradictory instructions have the opposite effect.

Diseases of occupations

Frank occupational disease is much less common today than fifty years ago. The expression 'as mad as a hatter' is evidence of the extremely high risk of mercury poisoning once faced by workers in the felt-hat industry, and many other occupational diseases were common enough to merit demotic names (knife-grinder's rot, potter's rot, painter's colic). Nevertheless, the old and long-recognized hazards continue to take toll of health and sometimes of life (in 1971 there were 89 cases of chrome ulceration, 123 of lead poisoning and four of mercurial poisoning), and many potentially harmful substances and processes are introduced into industry every year. To uncover new hazards and keep old ones under control there is need for frequent review of national mortality and morbidity data (Chapters 4 and 5), and for continual vigilance by occupational health workers.

A description, however brief, of all major occupational diseases would be out of place here. Recognition of the underlying industrial causes of some illnesses is part of clinical medicine, but too little attention is sometimes paid by doctors to the occupational background of their patients. Lead colic is still occasionally treated by appendicectomy, mercurialism dismissed as an anxiety state and the occupational origin of bladder cancer overlooked. Because the subject is so large we can provide only a short account of the ways in which harmful substances in the working environment may enter the body (this has important implications for prevention of occupational diseases), and mention only a few of the more important toxic dusts, fumes, vapours and gases encountered in industry.

(a) Portal of entry

Dusts, fumes, vapours and gases occur in great variety as industrial pollutants. Many of them are harmful to health, and it is not surprising that inhalation is the commonest way in which industrial disease is acquired. Some harmful pollutants act as simple asphyxiants: in this category are nitrogen (the blackdamp of mines), methane (firedamp) and carbon dioxide (found in fermentation vats and agricultural silos). Others act as chemical asphyxiants: carbon monoxide is very widely produced and used in industry and hydrogen sulphide (stink damp) is found in sewers and in mines. Many pollutants damage the respiratory passages: some have an immediately irritant effect (chlorine is used widely in the alkali industry and in dye works and paper mills, and ammonia is an important by-product of the gas and coke industry); some have an effect which does not become apparent until several hours after exposure (phosgene has many uses in the chemical industry);

others have a delayed and prolonged effect which is manifested as pneumoconiosis, numerically and socially still the most important industrial disease. Some atmospheric pollutants are absorbed from the respiratory passage into the blood, where they act as systemic poisons. This is the way in which lead, mercury, arsenic and cadmium poisoning are usually acquired, and some of the volatile organic compounds in common use in industry are powerful systemic poisons, acting on the central nervous system, blood-forming organs and liver and kidneys (carbon tetrachloride, trichlorethylene, tetrachlorethane, trinitro-toluene, benzene, methyl bromide, dichlorethylene and many others).

Some industrial poisons can penetrate the intact skin, but this mode of entry is uncommon. Aniline used in the dye industry (causing methaemoglobinaemia and liver and kidney damage), and organic phosphorus insecticides can be absorbed in this way.

Very occasionally an industrial poison enters the body by ingestion. Food is sometimes eaten in workrooms where lead or arsenic is being used, although this is prohibited by law; and industrial poisons, because they are readily available, are sometimes swallowed with suicidal intent. An often quoted example of disease due to ingestion of materials used at work occurred among girls applying radioactive paint to instrument dials in the United States during the First World War. Some of the girls who had made a habit of using their lips to get a good point on their paint brushes developed aplastic anaemia, necrosis of the jaw and bone cancer.

(b) The prescribed diseases

If persons working in specified occupations develop certain diseases, they become entitled to compensation under the National Insurance (Industrial Injuries) Act, 1946. These are the 'prescribed diseases'. Apart from pneumoconiosis, industrial disease is now uncommon, but it still occurs often enough for the clinician to bear it in mind when examining adult patients. The Schedule of Prescribed Diseases provides an indication of the continuing importance of industrial diseases and of the occupations with which they are known to be associated (table 24).

The distinction between 'prescribed' and 'notifiable' diseases is sometimes a source of confusion. The notifiable industrial diseases are as follows:

Table 24. Some examples of prescribed diseases

Disease or injury	Any occupation involving:
Poisoning by lead, manganese, phosphorus, arsenic, mercury, carbon bisulphide, benzene, nitro amino or chloro derivative of benzene, dinitrophenol, tetrachlorethane, tri-cresyl phosphate, tri-phenyl phosphate, diethylene dioxide (dioxan), methyl bromide, chlorinated naphthalene, nickel carbonyl, nitrous fumes, gonioma kamassi (African boxwood).	Use of, handling of, or exposure to fumes, dust or vapour of those substances or their homologues.
Anthrax.	Handling of wool, hair, bristles, hides, skins or animal products or residues, or contact with animals infected with anthrax.
Leptospira icterohaemorrhagica.	Work in rat-infested places.
Heat cataract.	Exposure to glare or rays from molten glass or molten red-hot metal.
Decompression sickness.	Work in compressed or rarified air.
Cramp of hand or forearm due to repetitive work.	Prolonged use of morse key. Prolonged writing. The twisting of cotton or woollen, including worsted yarn.
Traumatic inflammation of the tendons of the hand or forearm.	Manual labour involving frequent or repeated movements of the hand or wrist.
Poisoning by beryllium or its compounds.	Exposure to fumes, dust or vapour of beryllium.
Carcinoma of nasal mucous membrane or air sinus. Primary carcinoma of bronchus and lung.	Certain nickel procedures.
Tuberculosis.	Nursing, research work, laboratory worker, postmortem worker.

Table 24 (*continued*).

Disease or injury	Any occupation involving:
Primary neoplasm of the epithelial lining of the urinary bladder.	Exposure to alpha-naphthylamine or beta-naphthylamine, auramine or magenta and certain other compounds.
Cadmium.	Exposure to fumes of cadmium.
Non-infective dermatitis, excluding dermatitis due to ionizing particles and electromagnetic radiation.	Exposure to dust, liquid, or vapour.
Pulmonary disease due to the inhalation of the dust of mouldy hay or of other mouldy vegetable produce, and characterized by symptoms, and signs attributable to a reaction in the peripheral part of the broncho-pulmonary system, and giving rise to a defect in gas exchange (Farmer's lung).	Exposure to the dust of mouldy hay or other mouldy vegetable produce by reason of employment in: agriculture, horticulture or forestry; loading or unloading or handling in storage such hay or other vegetable produce; or handling bagasse.
Primary malignant neoplasm of the mesothelium (diffuse mesothelioma) of the pleura or of the peritoneum	The working or handling of asbestos or any admixture of asbestos; the manufacture or repair of asbestos textiles or other articles containing or composed of asbestos; the cleaning of any machinery or plant in any of the foregoing operations and of any chambers, fixtures and appliances for the collection of asbestos dust; substantial exposure to the dust arising from any of the foregoing operations.
Adeno-carcinoma of the nasal cavity or associated air sinuses.	Attendance for work in or about a building where wooden furniture is manufactured.
Pneumoconiosis and Byssinosis.	Special benefit in relation to a comprehensive list of occupations.

Lead poisoning	Epitheliomatous ulceration
Phosphorus poisoning	Chrome ulceration
Manganese poisoning	Carbon bisulphide poisoning
Arsenical poisoning	Aniline poisoning
Mercurial poisoning	Chronic benzene poisoning
Anthrax	Compressed air illness
Toxic jaundice	Toxic anaemia

All the notifiable diseases are also prescribed diseases but not all the prescribed diseases are notifiable. A doctor who finds that one of his patients has a notifiable disease has a statutory duty to notify the case to the Chief Inspector of Factories. The notification initiates an investigation of the occurrence with a view to preventing further cases.

CONTROL OF OCCUPATIONAL
HEALTH HAZARDS

Our short review of the influence of work on health suggests that control of health hazards in the working environment has two main aspects. The first is the need to protect the worker against dangerous substances, and since the respiratory tract is by far the commonest portal of entry to the body for industrial poisons, this above all requires control of atmospheric pollution. The second aspect is less precise, but not less important. It is to protect the worker against accident, and to control the physical environment—particularly the heat, light and noise—in which he works. We shall draw these two aspects of the problem together by considering five basic principles that apply to the control of all occupational hazards. Before stating the principles we must mention two of the aphorisms of Dr., later Sir Thomas Legge, the first medical inspector of factories.

1. Until the employer has done everything—and everything means a good deal—the workman can do next to nothing to protect himself although he is naturally willing enough to do his share.

2. If you can bring an influence to bear external to the workman (that is, one over which he can exercise no control), you will be successful—if you cannot or do not, you will never be wholly successful.

Legge's aphorisms imply that responsibility for control lies first and foremost with the employer: protective devices that depend for their use upon the 'will or whim of the worker to use them' (respirators, goggles, washing facilities) can never be completely effective. With this in mind we can list the first four principles for control of occupational health hazards in order of importance as: *substitution* (changing harmful materials and methods for safe ones); *isolation* (segregating dangerous processes, to reduce the opportunity for human contact); *ventilation* (drawing atmospheric pollutants away from the air workers are breathing); and *personal protection* (providing protective clothing and appliances for personal use). The fifth principle is *supervision*, without which none of the other principles can be applied.

Substitution

The fundamental approach to health hazards is to change harmful materials and methods for safe ones. The most effective method of dealing with an industrial poison is to use a non-toxic substance in its place. Two good historical examples are the substitution of red phosphorus and phosphorus sesquisulphide for white phosphorus in the manufacture of matches, which eradicated phosphorus necrosis of the jaw in workers in match factories, and the replacement of sandstone by carborundum grinding-wheels which played an important part in the control of silicosis. The substitution of wet for dry processes to suppress dust and of quiet for noisy typewriters in a large office to allay irritability are further examples of the application of this important principle.

Substitution is clearly the ideal means of eliminating or controlling a health hazard, but it is often the most difficult to put into practice. To introduce a safe for a dangerous substance may require extensive alterations in an industrial process. There may be no suitable substitute, and to find one may involve costly and protracted researches. In such circumstances most firms naturally prefer a less radical approach. However, substitution has the great advantage that in the last resort it can be enforced, by prohibiting the manufacture or use of a dangerous material. In this way ill health due to white phosphorus in the match industry, raw lead glazes in the pottery industry and 'silica flour' in foundries has been eliminated by statutory prohibition of those substances.

Isolation

If a dangerous process cannot be changed for a safer one, the obvious precaution is to isolate it so that few or no workers come into contact with it. This important principle is widely applied throughout industry. Toxic gases, poisonous fluids and harmful dusts are sealed off from the worker in retorts, pipes, ducts, flues, vats, tanks and stills. The complete enclosure of toxic substances may be a necessary part of an industrial process, as in much of the chemical industry, or it may be introduced to avoid waste or prevent explosion. Often it is the cheapest and most effective way of protecting workers against harmful atmospheric pollutants. However, even when toxic gases are completely enclosed, leaks may occur, causing danger for men working in the neighbour-hood. Carbon monoxide poisoning is a well recognized occupational hazard for blast furnace workers, and men cleaning and repairing closed systems are also at risk of accidental poisoning. Other applica-tions of the principle include segregating dangerous processes and materials in isolated buildings away from the main body of a works, transporting dangerous substances mechanically by means of enclosed conveyor belts and gravity feeds, handling radioactive isotopes by remote control, insulating noisy machinery, screening sources of radiant heat and fitting safety guards on dangerous machines.

Ventilation

Good ventilation adds greatly to the physiological and psychological comfort of people working indoors, whatever their occupations; it is essential to the health (and sometimes to the life) of people working in the neighbourhood of industrial processes which produce or use harm-ful dusts, mists, fumes or gases. In such circumstances good general ventilation, although it may reduce the hazard by diluting the toxic substances, is not enough. As we have seen, total enclosure of a process is the complete solution. But often this is not practicable, and the best safeguard is then a system of local exhaust ventilation to draw the harmful substances away from the air inhaled by workers and to carry it out of the workplace. When production of a dangerous substance is very localized (as it is in the case of grinding wheels and pneumatic chisels), high velocity ventilation through a small-bore duct with its opening close to the origin of the hazard is the solution. When atmo-spheric pollutants are produced over a wide area (as in foundries, steel-works and coal mines and in plating, pickling, galvanizing and paint-spraying workshops), the problem of their removal is technically much more difficult and may involve the design and installation of extensive and expensive extraction plant. Every industrial process presents its own problems, and often the atmospheric effluents need to be treated (by electrostatic precipitation, filtration, washing) before they can be discharged safely into the outside air.

Personal protection

In a few unusually dangerous working situations none of the above methods of control can be applied. For example, to rescue persons overcome by poisonous gases or to examine, repair or adjust enclosed processes men may have to enter and, for short periods, work in highly toxic atmospheres. The only satisfactory way to control such a dangerous situation is to provide the worker with personal safety appliances (for example, a self-contained breathing apparatus). In effect, this is an application of the isolation principle by enclosing the worker rather than the toxic process. Except in such uncommon circumstances, protective clothing and appliances should not be the first line defence against an unhealthy working environment. Although they are widely used in industry (dust respirators, goggles, helmets, safety shoes, gloves, barrier creams, ear plugs, chemical and fire resistant clothing) they should be regarded as no more than an extra precaution after the basic methods of controlling the environmental hazard have been applied. They can never be wholly satisfactory, for they depend for their effectiveness upon the cooperation of individual workers who may be careless. The appliances have the further disadvantage that they are often uncomfortable to wear and may interfere with movement, breathing or vision to the extent that they restrict a man's earning power.

Supervision

The four general principles referred to inevitably depend for their effective application upon supervision of the health of workers in relation to the environments in which they work. This can be carried out satisfactorily only by doctors, engineers, physicists and chemists with a special interest in occupational health. Doctors and occupational hygienists should be on the watch for the emergence of new hazards or the reappearance of old ones. Men and women at risk to known poisons need to be examined clinically at regular intervals (with appropriate laboratory tests) to ensure that their health is not being impaired (biological monitoring). The effectiveness of control of toxic and other hazards needs to be checked by routine environmental tests (environmental monitoring). Codes of safe practice are required and government inspection is necessary to ensure that employers comply with health and safety regulations.

OCCUPATIONAL HEALTH SERVICES

We shall now describe the occupational health services of Britain and comment on their effectiveness. From the time of Robert Owen many enlightened employers have carried their efforts to provide safe and healthy working conditions far beyond statutory requirements. But in general it is true to say that health supervision at work is one of the least satisfactory features of the country's health services. It is important to distinguish between statutory requirements and voluntary services.

Statutory requirements

Legislation about working conditions has a long history. It began with the Health and Morals of Apprentices Act (1802), which attempted to alleviate the pitiful condition of pauper children who were being sold from the poor law institutions of large cities to work in the mines and mills of the Midlands and North. It laid down that apprentices should not work for more than twelve hours a day (Saturdays included), that work rooms should be ventilated and that factory walls should be washed down twice a year. Seventeen years later the Factory Act, 1819, made it illegal to employ children who were less than nine years old. From these small beginnings a considerable body of legislation has developed. However, like so much of our social legislation, it has grown up piecemeal and the result often falls short of what is desirable and sometimes of what is clearly necessary. In particular, although the legislation is concerned for the most part only with minimum standards, the machinery devised to operate it is inadequate to ensure that even minimum standards are always observed.

The basic statutory provisions for control of the working environment and supervision of health and safety of workers are to be found in the Factories Act, 1961, and the Offices, Shops and Railway Premises Act, 1963. The statutory requirements fall into two broad groups, one concerned with general working conditions and the other with the more personal aspects of health and welfare.

(a) General working conditions

Workplaces must be kept clean and walls washed or painted as prescribed. Workrooms must not be overcrowded (a minimum of 40 square feet of floor space or 400 cubic feet of air space up to a height of ten feet per person), and they must be well ventilated (if necessary with local exhaust ventilation to protect workers against the inhalation of injurious atmospheric pollutants), suitably lighted and kept at a reasonable temperature (which should not be less than 60°F when a substantial part of the work done does not involve severe physical effort). Suitable seats must be provided for work that can be done sitting. There must be adequate facilities for accommodating and drying outdoor clothes and for washing (hot and cold water, soap and towels), a satisfactory supply of drinking water and a prescribed number of sanitary conveniences.

(b) Personal health and safety

Dangerous machinery must be securely fenced and effectively guarded, and hoists, lifts, cranes and lifting tackle must be sound and properly maintained, Meals must not be taken or meal times spent in rooms where poisons are used. Suitable goggles and other safety appliances must be provided in specified occupations, and special precautions must be taken against gassing and against explosion. A first aid box of the prescribed standard must be provided for every 150 persons employed and placed in charge of a responsible person with first aid training. Workers in certain prescribed occupations are also required to undergo periodic medical examination (for example, lead smelters, vitreous enamellers, tinners, mule spinners, and those working with ionizing radiations and with certain chemicals).

Employment Medical Advisory Service

Since February 1973 the Department of Employment has provided an Employment Medical Advisory Service to study and give advice about the medical problems related to people's work. The Service is headed by a Chief Medical Adviser with a small headquarters staff in London and a staff of about one hundred doctors (Employment Medical Advisers) with special knowledge of occupational health problems who are stationed in the main centres of industry. The service is designed to advise employers, employees, trade unions, general practitioners and others about the effects of particular jobs on health and to undertake medical examinations to protect employees against hazardous substances. It has special responsibilities in relation to young people whose school medical records indicate that they need to be careful in their choice of employment and in relation to the Department of Employment's placing, training and disablement resettlement services. It cooperates closely with H.M. Factory Inspectorate in ensuring that the health requirements of the Factories Act, 1961, are met and Employment Medical Advisers have right of entry to premises covered by the act, which prescribes penalties for obstructing Advisers.

Voluntary services

In recent years some of the large publicly controlled organizations (Coal Board, Steel Corporation, Dock Labour Board, Railways, London Transport, Post Office, Treasury), most of the large privately owned industries and an increasing number of small firms have begun to provide non-statutory occupational health services for their own employees. These services are paid for by the firms themselves and are quite independent of the Department of Employment services described above and of the National Health Service. At the present time about 650 doctors are employed as full-time industrial medical officers and a further 3,000 general practitioners as part-time officers in these health services. The services are essentially preventive in character, and at their best are designed to ensure that the health of workers is not impaired by their working environment and that workers are fit for and fitted to their work. They also provide first aid treatment for medical and surgical emergencies and continuing treatment for minor injuries and ailments; some of the larger organizations have set up dental, ophthalmic, orthopaedic, and chiropody clinics and some provide facilities for radiography and physiotherapy.

Present position

The two most unsatisfactory features of existing occupational health services are their uneven distribution and the inadequacy of laboratory facilities for examination and investigation of the working environment.

Apart from the advisory and supervisory services provided by the Department of Employment, nearly all occupational health services are non-statutory and paid for by the firms that provide them. As a result, large, wealthy and enlightened firms provide comprehensive services and small firms (where the worst working conditions often occur) provide little or nothing. In several areas services for groups of small factories are organized on a cooperative basis (for example at Slough, Harlow, Central Middlesex, Dundee, Rochdale, West Bromwich). But voluntary cooperation to provide non-statutory health and welfare services is not the answer to the national problem. Legal sanctions are needed, with a strengthened and greatly enlarged Factory Inspectorate to help employers to meet their statutory responsibilities.

In Britain laboratory facilities for recognizing and measuring harmful environmental influences at work are seriously deficient. Our services have fallen a long way behind those in the United States and compare unfavourably with those in most European countries. In recent years the Government has published many recommendations about threshold limit values (TLV) for toxic substances at place of work. But such recommendations lose much of their point if laboratory arrangements for measuring atmospheric concentration of the toxic substances are inadequate. At present the Department of Employment provides a limited public service, a few large firms employ their own occupational hygienists and occupational hygiene units in certain University Departments in London, Cardiff, Dundee, Manchester and Newcastle offer a problem-solving service for toxic and other environmental hazards.

FURTHER READING

Hunter D. (1969) *The Diseases of Occupations*, 4th Edition. English Universities Press, London.
Safety and Health at Work (1972) The Robens Report. H.M.S.O., London.

PART III

Services

19 · INTRODUCTION

EVOLUTION OF HEALTH SERVICES

It is useful to recognize four phases in the evolution of our health services. The first is the period before public responsibilities were accepted; the second is that in which public responsibilities developed; the third is the period of the National Health Service as originally planned; and the fourth is one in which there is a National Health Service modified in the light of about a quarter of a century's experience. With considerable differences in timing these phases can be recognized in the experience of other countries, although some have not yet entered the third phase of full acceptance of public responsibility for the finance and administration of services, and many have not even contemplated the fourth. That is to say, in most countries the health services provided or planned are still essentially of a traditional kind and nowhere have they been modified to the extent needed to bring them into line with modern requirements.

Phase 1, to 1848. Health services before public responsibility was accepted

It is not strictly true that there was no public responsibility for health services before the mid nineteenth century. Measures for quarantine and for isolation of the infectious had existed for centuries, and the destitute were admitted to county asylums after 1808 and to Poor Law institutions from 1834. But with these exceptions health services were financed by private or voluntary funds and the beginning of public services is usually and reasonably dated from the first Public Health Act of 1848. The history of health services before that time is essentially the history of hospitals and medical practice, discussed in Chapters 20 and 21 respectively.

Phase 2, 1848-1948. The development of public responsibility

The development of public responsibility for medical services in Britain before the introduction of the National Health Service covers a period of exactly one hundred years. It began with the introduction of environmental measures in 1848 and ended with acceptance of full responsibility for all preventive and therapeutic services in 1948. Approximately the first half of this period was concerned almost exclusively with control of communicable disease under local health authorities, mainly by environmental measures but including also provision of hospitals for infectious diseases. The year 1906 saw the extension of public services into the field of personal care (through the introduction of a school medical service), an extension restricted, however, to preventive medicine. In 1911 public responsibility was extended further into the field of treatment, by the National Health Insurance Act. This Act provided a limited service (essentially the services of a general practitioner and certain drugs) to some insured workers but not to their dependents. Finally, in 1948, the government introduced a comprehensive service, available to everyone, and financed mainly by taxation. The second phase is considered more fully in Chapter 22.

Phase 3, 1948-1974. The National Health Service

The National Health Service removed the burden of direct payment for medical services from the large number of people who could ill afford it and in the eyes of the general public this is probably its most considerable achievement. In doing so the Service did not interfere with the relationship between doctor and patient; nor did it prohibit private practice, although as a result of the provision of public services the volume of private work was inevitably reduced.

Indeed if the Service were to be criticized in the light of subsequent experience, the grounds would be, not that it departed from principles essential to the practice of medicine (a criticism sometimes made, particularly by visitors from countries which have not yet accepted a comprehensive public responsibility), but that it did not take the opportunity provided by public control to reorganize the services. Apart from the contraction of private care it made no significant change in the organization of medical practice; the public health service lost its responsibility for hospitals but was otherwise little affected; and while hospitals were brought under a new regional organization which eliminated the long-standing division between voluntary and public hospitals, the relationship of different types of hospitals to one another and to community health and welfare services remained essentially the same. However, while it is easy in retrospect it criticize the original organization of the National Health Service, it is questionable whether on the basis of the experience available in 1948 it would have been possible to do more.

Phase 4, from 1974. The reorganized National Health Service

It was not long after 1948 before it became evident that the traditional pattern of health services which had been incorporated with only minor modifications in the National Health Service was unsatisfactory. Perhaps the most obvious ground for criticism was that although the Ministry of Health (later the Department of Health and Social Security) was responsible for all parts of the Service, local and regional responsibility for general practitioner, hospital and local government services was divided between three administrative authorities. This led, *inter alia*, to duplication and deficiencies in services, and to an unfortunate division between community and hospital and between preventive and therapeutic medicine. The changes introduced from 1974 were intended to eliminate these divisions, by establishing a unified district, area and regional organization with the responsibility and power to plan comprehensively the health services required by a defined population.

The National Health Service and its reorganization in 1974 are discussed in Chapter 24.

THE BACKGROUND OF PRESENT DAY SERVICES

Until the nineteenth century, medical measures comprised no more than the service of doctors to sick patients, and even today, when there has been more than a hundred years' experience of preventive medicine, the original concept is still deeply rooted in public and professional consciousness as the essential medical role. This is what brings most students into medicine and it largely determines the character of medical education and the direction of medical science and service. However the traditional concept is beginning to be re-examined, and the present time may prove to be of outstanding importance in the history of medicine as the first in which the requirements for health and the nature of the medical task were seen in perspective. At least three influences are contributing to this reappraisal: the changing character of health problems; the growth of technology; and acceptance of comprehensive public responsibility for provision of medical services.

The change in health problems

If a biologist who had given no special thought to the determinants of human health were invited to express an opinion about them, his reasoning might be along the following lines. Throughout his existence man, like other living things, has been exposed to a high risk of disease and death. In technologically developed countries, this risk has greatly diminished, largely as a result of medical measures, particularly those directed to the prevention and treatment of disease in the individual. In consequence, the health problems of today are different from those of the past; but since medical science will continue to advance, the problems also must be expected to change. Moreover, they will do so in ways which cannot be foreseen, for neither the pace nor the direction of scientific progress can be predicted for more than very short periods.

Such an interpretation would be mistaken both in its emphasis on specific medical measures and in regarding the change in health problems as essentially a continuum. The experience of the past two centuries, discussed in Chapters 1 and 2, indicates that the main influences on health are not the prevention and treatment of disease in the individual; and, although health will continue to change, there is nevertheless an important distinction to be made between the problems of the past and those of the foreseeable future. Indeed, the twentieth century may come to be recognized as a watershed separating the infectious diseases which have been predominant during man's evolution from the residual problems which remain when infections are reduced to small proportions. These are particularly congenital handicaps, mental illness, and the disease and disability associated with ageing, problems in which, in general, medical research has been least interested and medical services least successful. Changes in the residual problems are of course inevitable, but it is unlikely that we shall see ever again a change in the spectrum of disease as profound as that which resulted from the decline of infections.

The growth of technology

A second influence on thinking about health is the increasing cost of medical services, due largely to the spectacular and, in its financial and administrative implications, alarming advance of technology. Until the nineteenth century there were few methods of investigating and treating diseases, and even in the first part of the present century, their number was relatively small. In the past few decades, however, there has been an enormous increase in the volume and complexity of technology in medicine and there can be no doubt that it will continue, probably at an increasing rate. The growth of technology is largely responsible for rising costs which result not only from expensive equipment and facilities but from the heavy demands on technical and professional staff. It is not possible to envisage the level of development of technology by the end of the century, but long before then it is likely that its complexities and costs will have exposed the inadequacies of the traditional research and service matrix and forced the consideration of cost benefit and priorities in medicine which doctors and their patients are still reluctant to contemplate.

Public responsibility

A third influence is acceptance of public responsibility for the finance and administration of health services which in most developed countries is now extensive or complete. For the first time it is both possible and necessary to examine the medical scene as a whole, to consider the balance between research and practice, between prevention and treatment, between care and cure. Medical services can no longer ignore related social services, hospitals cannot function without reference to domiciliary and ambulatory care, and traditional public health needs to be reshaped in relation to the greatly enlarged public commitment for medical services.

Each of these influences, changed problems, technological advance, and public responsibility, is important; but it is their coincidence which makes it imperative to reconsider the framework of medical services. The public commitment has come at a time when the outstanding problems are in general more intractable than those they have replaced and when elaborate methods threaten to stretch the resources of even the wealthiest countries. Serious mistakes in organization will be penalized more heavily than in the past, and it is therefore essential to devise a new pattern in accord with the character of the residual health problems and the trend in medical technology.

LIMITATION OF COSTS: MEDICAL PRIORITIES

One of the most formidable problems confronting health services is to find some rational basis of restricting costs which are already high and appear to be potentially unlimited. An international study of health expenditure made for the World Health Organization in 1967 showed that some countries are now spending over 6 per cent of the gross national product on health services, and if present trends continue the proportion will rise to 10 per cent before the end of the century. No country is so wealthy that it can afford to be indifferent to the need to restrict expenditure on health services.

If costs are not to be restricted on an arbitrary basis, there will have to be a new development in medical accounting and a system of priorities. This raises four questions: Are priorities necessary? How can they be reconciled with the obligations of the doctor to his patient? Who should decide priorities? On what basis can they be determined? There is as yet no answer to these questions, which are only beginning to receive the attention they deserve.

Are medical priorities necessary?

Reactions to the imposition of prescription charges in the National Health Service some years ago indicated that many people find the whole idea of medical priorities distasteful. They see the need to curtail other public activities, including social services, and recognize that this requires a choice between alternative policies according to their cost and usefulness. Medical services, however, are quite another matter; it is hard to accept suffering from disease due, not to lack of knowledge of prevention or cure, but to insufficient resources to provide essential services. This reaction, though understandable, is based on certain misconceptions which need to be removed if medical priorities are to be considered rationally.

First, it should be recognized that potential medical expenditure is unlimited, an anomaly to which both the public and doctors contribute in different ways. On the one hand, the public appetite for medical services appears to be insatiable. Just as any child can occupy the attention of as many adults as are willing to look after it, some patients seem able to absorb the time of all the doctors who can be persuaded to see them; and in hospitals, with Parkinsonian logic, patients appear to increase in number to fill the available beds. On the other hand, many doctors are reluctant to consider effectiveness and costs, and vigorously defend their right to make up their minds about what is good for their patients without regard for such tiresome criteria. The surgeon who operated on the tuberculous back or chest did not often consider that it would have been cheaper, more humane and more effective to improve housing or prohibit the sale of infected milk; and the psychoanalyst does not inquire whether the results of his therapy are commensurate with the long hours he and his patient spend in communion. All that is necessary to satisfy public scrutiny or private conscience is to ensure that a procedure is well intended and has some claim to consideration, at least in the judgement of the doctor who uses it. In such circumstances, it is clearly impossible to set limits on expenditure.

A second source of misunderstanding is the belief that the assignment of priorities in medicine would introduce a new principle. In fact, they are already well established; it never has been possible to do all the things which could usefully be done if there were no limits to resources, and in underdeveloped countries in Asia, Africa and Latin America the practical possibilities are restricted to a small fraction of those which knowledge would justify. Very often, however, the choice between alternative measures is made on quite inadequate grounds and with little reference to medical objectives.

A further misconception is that health depends mainly on treatment of the sick, and that any reduction in the volume of curative services would have disastrous consequences. Interpretation of the reasons for human health leads to quite a different conclusion: the most important influences are an adequate diet and avoidance of environmental hazards such as contaminated food, infected water, polluted air, and tobacco. If health is to be placed on a different footing from other social goals, concern about restriction of expenditure should not be limited to medicine, but should logically be extended to other social services such as nutrition and housing. There are also no grounds for undue concern about the consequences of some restriction on treatment services. Indeed, it is questionable whether there is any method of treatment of which it could be said confidently that a substantial increase in investment would lead to a commensurate improvement in health in Britain. This claim could be made for some environmental measures, such as elimination of atmospheric pollution and improved nutrition.

How can priorities be reconciled with the doctor's obligations to his patient?

Two examples will illustrate the difficulty in reconciling the interests of society with the doctor's obligations to his patient. In Britain about, six in every thousand children are born with a serious malformation of the central nervous system. Those with the most lethal abnormality, anencephalus, are stillborn or die soon after delivery, so that unless some dextrous but misguided surgeon finds the means of prolonging life in the absence of a brain, the problem will not extend beyond birth. Most children with the other common conditions, such as spina bifida and hydrocephalus, also die within a few years, but the proportion surviving, although still small, can be increased by surgical intervention. However, surgery does not often restore normal functions; most children who survive as a result of it are paralyzed to some degree for the rest of their lives, and the degree of paralysis can usually be predicted at the time of operation. Some are also mentally retarded. If the most active surgical measures were practiced on every viable child with spina bifida, the number disabled by this condition would be approximately trebled, and a substantial increase in places in special schools would be required. On the two most important points the malformations of the central nervous system differ from some others, notably those of the heart: operation on a cardiac malformation may restore a child to normal health, and even when it is unsuccessful it does not increase the number who survive with a serious handicap.

A very different example of a possible conflict between the aims of society and those of the individual is in the field of family planning. Control of population growth is a necessary condition for human health. Even in technologically advanced countries such as Britain, population size is already too great and, from a public viewpoint, it is at the least irresponsible to have a large family. Yet for understandable reasons, the family planning movement operates as a service, not to the community but to individuals, providing them with knowledge and methods that will enable them to have the number of children they desire.

Is it possible to reconcile such diverse private and public ends? No mother would feel safe in bringing her malformed child to a doctor for surgery if she thought his first concern was the public consequence of his action; and the demand for family planning services might soon decline if it were known that in the view of the clinic staff, families having more than about two children were socially irresponsible. Yet, if these personal services are to have no regard for public goals, what is to prevent a large increase in the number of handicapped people, and how is population size to be kept in some reasonable relation to national resources?

Perhaps the first point to be made is that these are medical issues only to the extent that the doctor provides the information on which the decision is based and is often the agent by whom it is implemented. The primary right of decision is the patient's or, in the case of the malformed child who cannot act for himself, the parents'. This is true when the doctor advises the parents, or even when he is in effect asked to decide for them, as he usually is, for example when a mother is confronted by the impossible choice between short term risk and long term cure from an operation on her child with a malformed heart. In some respects the doctor's position is analogous to that of the barrister who tries to act for his client as his client would act for himself, if he had the requisite knowledge and experience.

The doctor's position is, however, more complicated than that of the barrister in that there are considerable differences of medical opinion about appropriate and justifiable methods of treatment. Since these differences are determined more by religious and moral than by professional convictions, they must be respected. It would surely be wrong to require a doctor to refuse treatment to a patient he believes he can help. What can be asked is that before making his decision the doctor should inform himself about its medical and social consequences. If there are grounds for dissatisfaction with the present position they are that medical opinion is often ill-informed rather than that it is not uniform.

If, however, the doctor is to be free to decide the method of treatment, what can prevent the imposition of an intolerable burden on the medical and social services? The answer, so far as there is one, lies not in directives to the doctor but in the disposition of medical resources. If Freudian psychiatrists are sent to Botswana, they must be expected to practice psychoanalysis. The individual physician has to answer the question: 'Shall I refuse to help my patient?' For society as a whole, however, the question takes the more tractable form: 'How best can medical resources be deployed?' It is understandable that a surgeon may find it impossible to refuse to correct a cardiac malformation in a Mongol child brought to him for assistance. However, in establishing national priorities in the use of medical manpower, the medical and social consequences should be taken into account, and they would undoubtedly show that there are more urgent requirements than thoracic units in mental subnormality hospitals. Such a decision cannot reasonably be criticized as a denial of life to the handicapped, and if the time ever comes when resources are sufficient for all purposes, the formidable problem of medical priorities will no longer arise.

Who should decide priorities?

If the main burden of assessing priorities is to be removed from the practicing doctor, who, on behalf of society, is to take it up? The assessment is best made where major decisions are taken concerning the disposition of resources, and in Britain most are at national, regional or local level. This discussion will be limited to centrally determined priorities.

The central government department already makes many decisions about priorities. It determines the allocation of resources to different services and regions; and even within regions it has a large influence on the way money is spent. Yet in spite of this close supervision of expenditure, there is considerable hesitation in establishing national policies. There is particular reluctance to do anything from the centre that might be interpreted as interference with the doctor's judgement concerning the best treatment for his patient.

With due regard for these reservations, there are nevertheless some issues on which it is inconceivable that a large number of regional and local authorities will all arrive at wise, well informed and, where necessary, consistent policies, and in respect of which it seems essential to consider priorities at the centre. Mechanisms for doing so already exist, but they need to be developed and in some cases modified in relation to particular problems.

On what basis can medical priorities be determined?

The last is perhaps the most difficult of the four issues. All that will be attempted here is a brief comment on two important criteria; effectiveness and efficiency.

Among the first questions to be asked about a medical procedure is whether it is effective for the purpose—prevention, diagnosis or treatment—for which it is employed. This is different from the question of efficiency discussed below, for it asks only whether a procedure is effective, without reference to its costs or the possible alternative uses of the same resources.

There is no doubt about the need to assess the effectiveness of medical methods, both those which may be introduced and many that are already in use. Oliver Wendell Holmes said that if all our drugs were thrown into the Pacific Ocean it would be so much the better for mankind and so much the worse for the fishes. The position is somewhat better today, but there are still a good many procedures of which the best that can be said is that they have not been shown to be effective in the circumstances in which they are employed.

This position is clearly unsatisfactory, but it has this excuse: the problems associated with evaluation of effectiveness in medicine are often quite formidable. In some cases they require not only assessment of a diagnostic or therapeutic method, but also extension of knowledge of the natural history of disease that may require investigation of a large population over many years. In judging the value of screening for cancer of the cervix, for example, it is not enough to show that the recognition of abnormal cells makes it possible to detect carcinoma *in situ*. It is also necessary to know the frequency with which carcinoma *in situ* progresses to invasive cancer. For these among other reasons, the assessment of medical priorities requires a considerable extension of research into the effectiveness of medical procedures.

When a procedure is shown to be effective, and logically not before, the question arises whether it deserves to replace alternative methods which are already in use or might be introduced. This takes medical research into the difficult study of efficiency, for which techniques of cost/benefit analysis have been developed in other fields of applied science. It is clearly distinguished from the appraisal of effectiveness, being concerned not merely with whether a procedure is useful, but also with whether it makes better use of the resources required than the alternatives available.

Such a decision is most readily reached when both costs and benefits can be quantified. In medicine it is conceivable that costing might be put on a satisfactory numerical basis, although even this would not be easy. There have been few attempts to determine the costs of individual medical procedures and there is not yet a consistent basis which takes account of the large number of contributing influences commonly involved. For example, hospitals do not dissect the cost of, say, thoracic surgery from other expenditure; nor do they estimate accurately in the field of thoracic surgery the cost of removing a cancerous lung.

But it is the appraisal of benefit which raises the greatest difficulties. Some indices may be of use for specific and limited purposes: for example the duration of stay in hospital and, in the case of working adults, the amount of time lost from work. However, there are important benefits which cannot be quantified in this way. Indeed the goal of reducing all medical benefits to a common quantitative basis is almost certainly illusory, and the final decision between alternatives must usually rest on a value judgement. Nevertheless this judgement should be based on much fuller and more accurate information than in the past, information about costs and benefits, quantified to the extent that this is possible but also amplified by other kinds of evidence.

FURTHER READING

ABEL-SMITH B. (1967) *An International Study of Health Expenditure*. World Health Organization, Geneva, Switzerland.

COCHRANE, A. L. (1972) *Effectiveness and Efficiency*. Oxford University Press for The Nuffield Provincial Hospitals Trust, London.

MCKEOWN T. (1965) *Medicine in Modern Society*. George Allen and Unwin Ltd., London.

MCLACHLAN G. (ed.) (1971) *Challenges for Change*. Oxford University Press for the Nuffield Provincial Hospitals Trust, London.

MCLACHLAN G. and MCKEOWN T. (eds.) (1971) *Medical History and Medical Care*. Oxford University Press for the Nuffield Provincial Hospitals Trust, London.

EVOLUTION OF HEALTH AND RELATED SOCIAL SERVICES

20 · HOSPITALS

The earliest hospitals were religious institutions concerned mainly with the care of the destitute. Few of them survived the suppression of the monasteries in the sixteenth century, and for 300 years there was little institutional provision for the sick. In 1700 there were less than a dozen hospitals in the country, of which about half were in London. Soon after that date several voluntary hospitals were founded, and large numbers were added during the next two centuries.

The voluntary hospitals were secular organizations supported by charity, and in the beginning their purpose was to continue the work of the Church by caring for the sick and needy. However, in the late seventeenth century St Thomas's began to restrict admissions to short term cases. This practice was soon followed by other hospitals, and it became necessary to find other accommodation for the patients excluded. They comprised the destitute sick, the mentally ill, the infectious, sick children and pregnant women.

Provision was made for some of these classes in specialized voluntary hospitals, and this explains the separation of many children's, women's and special hospitals from general hospitals. But three large classes— the mentally ill, the destitute sick and the infectious—were beyond the resources, and to some extent outside the interest, of the voluntary movement. It was therefore necessary to make public provision for them.

The first important public development was the founding of county asylums for pauper lunatics in 1808. In retrospect this can be seen as a significant step, since it separated the hospital care of the mentally ill from general hospitals. In 1889 the asylums were transferred to the new county and county borough councils, which remained responsible until 1948 when the National Health Service Act placed all hospitals under a common administration.

The next major step in development of public hospitals followed the Poor Law Amendment Act of 1834, which made it necessary for those receiving public assistance to enter a workhouse. It was not intended to provide hospital accommodation; but many destitute people admitted to Poor Law institutions were sick, and this led to the establishment of a second public hospital system, separate from both the voluntary general and the public mental hospitals.

The results could hardly have been more unsatisfactory. The beds in mixed workhouses were unsuitable for the care of the sick. Medical supervision was by badly paid part-time general practitioners, and the nursing by pauper inmates. In 1867 Parliament authorized the construction of infirmaries, designed as hospitals and intended to provide a more acceptable standard of care. Unfortunately the infirmaries soon followed the practice of the voluntary hospitals and began to exclude patients requiring prolonged care. This left the ill-equipped asylums and Poor Law hospitals with most of the work for the mentally ill and the sick poor.

A third division of the public hospital service resulted from concern about infectious disease. The voluntary hospitals did not accept most infectious patients, and stimulated by the appearance of cholera in Britain, Parliament authorized the construction of fever hospitals by local authorities in 1867. From this time there were four hospital systems, one voluntary and three public: asylums, later called mental hospitals; Poor Law hospitals for the destitute sick; and hospitals for the infectious. In 1929 the hospital responsibilities of the Poor Law were transferred to the major local authorities, and in 1948 the National Health Service Act placed all hospitals, voluntary and public, under the Ministry of Health.

This brief account of the early development of hospitals explains the origin of many of their present difficulties. It shows that this most complex of social services was essentially unplanned, and owes its character largely to a series of arbitrary decisions taken by voluntary and public administrations. Even the elementary question of the numbers and types of beds needed to serve a population was never considered seriously. The important issue of the relationship between different types of hospitals was completely ignored. The restrictive policy of the voluntary hospitals, adopted also by the public infirmaries, led to the separate general hospital. The county asylums, founded to care for one of the large classes of patients rejected by the voluntary movement, were the forerunners of the separate mental hospital. And the relegation of the destitute sick to the workhouses brought about the isolation of the chronic hospital.

HOSPITALS TODAY

The failure to plan hospitals is still reflected in the services of most countries. Hospitals may have less than 50 beds or more than 2,000; their sites vary in size from a few to several hundred acres. They may be located in industrial, commercial, rural or residential areas. There are large hospitals where there are few people and large numbers of people where there are few hospitals. Teaching hospitals are established with no clearly defined relationship to other hospitals, even to other teaching hospitals in the same area, and the division between the major classes of hospitals—acute, chronic, mental illness and subnormality—are still determined largely by the circumstances in which they developed. There are still no satisfactory answers to fundamental questions concerning hospital size, location and function.

The absence of planning which is evident in the distribution of hospitals is also seen in the use of their sites. Many are too small to provide scope for essential development; and good sites are often spoiled by failure to plan imaginatively, allowing for growth and change of use of facilities.

It can hardly be doubted that the role of hospitals will be more complex in future than in the past. At least three major influences are at work: the increasing sophistication of methods of investigating and treating disease; the complexity of the medical problems which have resulted from the decline of infectious disease; and the fact that in technologically advanced countries hospitals are becoming the focal point of medical activities. If hospitals are to meet the many demands on them their development must no longer be determined by ephemeral circumstances but planned with due regard for long-term objectives. Three fundamental issues are their integration, size and relation to welfare services.

Integration of hospital services

We have noted that the separation of the major classes of hospitals resulted from restriction of the work of the voluntary general hospitals, and from division of public responsibility for mental, destitute and infectious patients. The results have been deplorable, both in their effect on the standards of care of patients, and in their far-reaching influence on hospital development. The following are some of the consequences of fragmentation of responsibility.

(a) *Mixing of patients with different needs.* The patients in mental, chronic and acute hospitals are not homogeneous in respect of their medical, nursing and social needs. Patients in mental and chronic hospitals may exhibit the full range of physical and mental illness; some of them are indistinguishable clinically from others in general hospitals. Mental hospitals have patients who do not require psychiatric care and chronic hospitals have patients who do. All three classes of hospitals have some patients who should not be in hospital at all.

(b) *Division of patients into acute and chronic classes.* The traditional segregation of hospitals gives the erroneous impression that in their need for care patients divide naturally into acute and chronic classes. This impression results from the reluctance of acute hospitals to admit or retain patients who will occupy a bed for more than a few weeks, and from the deficient services of mental and chronic hospitals, particularly in the acute phase of illness. With adequate care at all stages of illness the distribution of duration of stay in hospital would look quite different.

(c) *Staffing difficulties.* Probably the most difficult problem confronting mental, chronic and subnormality hospitals is that of attracting doctors and nurses in sufficient numbers. It will remain unsolved so long as these hospitals are isolated from the mainstream of medical and nursing interest represented by the general hospital.

(d) *Inflexibility.* It is essential that hospitals should respond to changes in the demands for care and in methods of investigation and treatment. In part this capacity for change is determined by internal construction and site planning; but it is also influenced profoundly by the location of the major divisions of the service. So long as hospitals are isolated from one another they must be inherently inflexible, for it is then much more difficult to convert unwanted facilities to alternative use, and to transfer redundant staff to different work.

(e) *Uneconomic construction and operation.* An isolated hospital must be largely self-sufficient, since it cannot readily exploit complementary services of other hospitals. This affects both construction and operation:

capital costs are higher, because each hospital must have its own surgical, radiological, laboratory and other facilities, and because these facilities are not used fully, operating costs are inevitably increased.

In order to avoid the disadvantages of isolation it has been suggested that in future hospitals should be planned with the following features:

1. All types of patients should be cared for at a common centre in approximately the proportions in which they occur in the related population.

2. Patients should be classified according to their medical, nursing and other needs and placed in the facilities most suitable for their care.

3. In view of the wide range of patients' needs, the hospital should consist of a number of buildings, with varied size, design, equipment and staff.

4. Medical and nursing services should be provided by a common staff.

A hospital centre incorporating these features has been referred to as a balanced hospital community.

The idea of assembling a number of hospital buildings on the same site is not new. Architects and hospital planners have often been attracted by the possibilities of centres providing multiple buildings with some centralized services, and in the period between the two World Wars several were established. Moreover there are places in Britain where, for historical reasons, chronic, mental and general hospitals were built near to one another. But such hospital centres have not departed from the traditional view of the role of the hospital, for in spite of their location on the same or adjoining sites the hospitals remained single units, separately staffed and with independent services.

Because it is concerned with all classes of patients, the balanced hospital would have its greatest impact on psychiatric, geriatric and subnormal patients who have suffered most from past deficiencies. On the same site, with a common staff, the standard of care could be raised to a level long considered obligatory in general hospitals. Moreover, the end of isolation would contribute largely to a change in public attitudes to mental and chronic illness.

But although the impact of the balanced hospital community would be greatest on psychiatric and geriatric care, all parts of the hospital service would be affected in some degree. For example, paediatrics requires a close association with obstetrics in investigation of prenatal influences, with general medicine and surgery in exploitation of methods of investigation and treatment, and with psychiatry in consideration of the psychologically disturbed child. Even for general medical and surgical services, which are well developed in many hospitals, there would be considerable advantages in proximity, for example in the possibility of immediate transfer of patients who no longer need acute care to a more appropriate unit.

If a hospital is to respond to future requirements it must be designed to allow for growth, change of use and replacement. These are essentially matters for the architect. With a spacious site and imaginative planning it should be possible for a hospital to meet the needs of a defined population over a long period.

Not the least of the advantages of the balanced hospital would be the opportunity to improve its appearance. The contemporary hospital is still a forbidding structure which introduces patients and relatives into an alien world. Particularly for those who are ambulant, and whose stay is measured in months rather than days, the general character of the centre is important. The aim should be a domestic rather than an institutional appearance over a substantial part of the site. It can be achieved by reducing the scale of the buildings, by variation of structure and design, and by separation of hospital facilities by other amenities such as shops and restaurants, needed by a considerable resident population.

Hospital size

Many hospitals, including some planned recently, are too small to make economic use of expensive technological methods whose efficient operation requires a large input. Such methods, and the more elaborate ones which will undoubtedly follow, make it desirable either to centralize the services for several hospitals or to build larger hospitals. There are several reasons for preferring the latter approach.

Most hospitals are also unable to provide a full range of specialist experience. It has been estimated that six physicians and six surgeons are needed for this purpose, and when numbers of other types of consultants are increased proportionately, the hospital is capable of serving a population of more than 250,000. It is difficult to predict the number of beds required in a hospital of this kind, working closely with well developed community services, but by present day British standards it would have about 2,000. Of course, there must be variation in hospital size and function according to the density of population served.

In opposition to the trend towards increased size, it has been suggested that the large hospital will be too far from patients and difficult to administer. The problem of distance would not arise in most urban areas, and in Britain over 90 per cent of the population would be less —usually much less—than 15 to 20 miles from a major hospital. Compromises are needed in rural areas, and they can be of various kinds: hospitals smaller than would, in general, be desirable; greater distances for patients and relatives to travel; and provision of local facilities, possibly for long-stay geriatric or psychiatric patients, who ideally should not be separated from the main hospital.

All large institutions have administrative problems; but they are not insuperable, and in other fields such as industry and universities they have not been allowed to stand in the way of expansion where this was thought to be justified on other grounds.

Relation between hospital and welfare services

For some time it has been evident that many psychiatric, geriatric and mentally subnormal patients are in the wrong place. Some are at home or in welfare homes although they need hospital care; others are in acute or psychiatric hospitals when they no longer need their services; still others remain in geriatric and subnormality hospitals only because they have no home to which they can return.

Two recent investigations showed the extent of the problem in Britain. In the first it was found that, on the assumption that only those needing hospital investigation and treatment or continuous care from a trained nursing staff should be in the hospital, approximately 50 per cent of patients in hospitals for the mentally retarded are misplaced. The transfer of such patients to their homes with supporting services, or to hostels under local authorities, is essential if the hospital problems presented by the retarded are to be reduced to manageable proportions. The transfer is also in the interest of those who do not need hospital services, since they may not get the necessary educational training and occupational opportunities under a medical administration.

The second inquiry was concerned with geriatric patients in hospitals, seeking admission to hospitals, or in welfare homes. The results again showed a substantial overlap of functions: some patients were in hospitals although they did not require their services whereas others for whom hospital care was desirable were seeking admission or were in welfare homes.

It is a valid criticism of the National Health Service that it has not yet come to terms with this problem of misplacement of patients, a problem which is due largely to the fact that the respective responsibilities of hospital and welfare authorities have not been clearly defined. It is admittedly not always easy to say whether a patient requires hospital care, for the decision cannot be based on the nature of the disabilities, which are continuously graded from trivial to serious. However the distinction can usually be made by focusing attention on the types of care required, and in such borderline cases it is the need for continuous nursing which makes it desirable for a patient to be in hospital. In practice it is usually not difficult to decide whether a patient's mental or physical condition makes it necessary for him to be under the care of trained staff.

THE TEACHING CENTRE

We shall now consider the bearing of the balanced hospital concept on medical education and the teaching hospital. Some people would say is has no bearing at all. They believe the traditional centre is admirably suited to its three-fold obligation: to provide service of the highest quality; to teach; and to do research.

Patients admitted to teaching hospitals are highly selected, although this is truer of some services than of others. For example geriatrics and psychiatry, are either excluded altogether, or represented by small numbers of beds which bear little relation to the actual size of the problems. Other services, such as those concerned with diseases of the ear, nose and throat may be disproportionately large.

It is not difficult to understand how the restrictions arose; they resulted from grafting the concept of scientific medicine on the tradition of voluntary hospitals. From the time of its rebirth in the eighteenth century, the work of voluntary hospitals was sharply restricted. Those providing voluntary funds were entitled to decide how they should be used, and medical staff receiving little or no remuneration could reasonably expect to determine the nature of the work. Both interests coincided in agreement to leave to the State the problems of mental illness, mental subnormality, infectious disease, and all types of infirmity associated with destitution.

The selectiveness of teaching centres has been accentuated in the twentieth century by the interests of scientific medicine. The unexceptionable wish to make medical schools centres of research led inevitably to selection of patients in respect of whom knowledge was advancing. They did not include the mentally ill or the chronic sick, who were thus removed from the experience of students and the minds of research workers.

But if the teaching hospital is not characteristic of all hospitals, it is even less representative of medical care as a whole. It has no responsibility for domiciliary services, and is quite divorced from the health work of local authorities. Some medical schools attempt to remedy these deficiencies by sending students to general practitioners and to local authority clinics. Nevertheless it is still true that the teaching hospital presents only a restricted view of the institutional care of selected patients.

These restrictions are usually defended on two grounds. First, it is suggested they are needed in order to put before students a high level of clinical practice. And second, for research it is thought desirable to focus attention on diseases of which knowledge is advancing. The limitation of work has, however, three serious disadvantages: one in the effect on medical education; another in respect of medical organization; and a third in relation to medical research.

It is widely recognized that doctors acquire their concept of practice largely from clinical teachers and often leave the teaching hospital hoping to do the kind of work they saw as students. Since this excludes responsibility for large classes of patients and is based on the most sophisticated methods, it provides an inadequate preparation for many of the realities of practice.

A second objection is that teaching centres are prevented from contributing to thought about the way in which medical knowledge is applied; indeed the contemporary organization of research finds little place for concern with services. Yet the problems raised by the application of medical knowledge are at least as formidable as those associated with its acquisition, and are unlikely to be solved unless taken seriously at teaching centres.

A third disadvantage is that the restrictions limit the scope of research, since they remove important diseases from the observation and experience of the investigator. The slow progress with mental deficiency and schizophrenia must be due in part to their exclusion in the past from teaching hospitals. Moreover there are many medical problems which require study of representative patients from known populations. In most teaching centres it is impossible to identify the population from which patients are derived.

To remedy these deficiencies it would be necessary for teaching hospitals to accept responsibility for exploring new patterns of practice. They should do so both because they can make an important contribution to the development of services, and because the demonstration of a modern concept of practice is essential to the education of students.

Perhaps the simplest way of creating the right environment is to accept responsibility for all institutional services of an area, preferably the one in which the teaching hospital is placed. This would ensure access to all patients from a defined population. But it is also necessary to break down the barriers between institutional and domiciliary medical care and between preventive and therapeutic medicine. For these purposes it would be desirable to associate the teaching centre with all the services in the area.

We have discussed the advantages of a defined population in which responsibility is accepted for all patients. But teaching hospitals are also engaged in service, teaching and research of a more specialized kind, for which it is necessary to admit a substantial number of selected patients. A well planned teaching centre would achieve a balance between the two activities: a comprehensive service to a local population; and a service to selected patients drawn from a much wider area.

21 · MEDICAL PRACTICE

It is useful to distinguish three periods in the history of medical practice. Until the eighteenth century there were no consultants and practitioners as we now know them, and services were provided by physicians, surgeons and apothecaries. The physician was a professional man, trained in a university and his practice was restricted to a small wealthy clientele. The surgeon was a craftsman, trained by apprenticeship; his work was supposed to be limited to surgical procedures, but many surgeons also practised midwifery, kept shops and dispensed drugs. The least considered of the medical workers was the apothecary, a tradesman trained by apprenticeship, who was allowed to charge only for the sale of drugs prescribed by physicians. But by the seventeenth century apothecaries were seeing patients and writing prescriptions and, unacknowledged, they had become the doctors of the middle and poorer classes.

The second period dates from the eighteenth century when, with the founding of voluntary hospitals, the distinctions between physician, surgeon and apothecary began to disappear. It became important to a doctor to have a hospital appointment, and a new division was established between those who had and those who had not. From this time the status of the surgeon improved, and some apothecaries began to work in hospitals.

The third period began with the 1858 Medical Act. By preparing the way for common recruitment, training and registration of doctors it finally removed the historical distinction between physician, surgeon and apothecary. But by this time the new, and from a present day viewpoint more significant, distinction between consultant and practitioner was well established. It was based, not on substantial differences in training or competence, but on hospital appointments. The British Medical Journal described the country consultant as 'the general practitioner who owes his position to the fact of his holding an appointment in connection with a country hospital.'

We have already discussed the deficiencies of medical services which at the beginning of the century led to the suggestion that there should be a public medical service. This proposal was not accepted, and the only public provision for the care of the sick outside hospital was through the medical officers employed by the Poor Law. In 1911, however, a Liberal Government, with Lloyd George as Chancellor of the Exchequer, introduced a scheme of National Health Insurance financed by compulsory deductions from wages. This method had been used in Europe from about 1883; but the proposal was criticized in Britain by workers and employers who objected to contributions from wages and profits, and by some doctors who disliked even a limited degree of state control. Nevertheless the National Health Insurance Act had the support of public opinion and of many doctors who were satisfied that under it they would be better off.

The Act provided for insured workers the domiciliary services of a general practitioner and some drugs. It did not include hospital or consultant care, and made no provision for dependants. These deficencies were the main reasons for dissatisfaction with National Health Insurance, and led in 1948 to its replacement by a comprehensive service.

THE ORGANIZATION OF MODERN PRACTICE

The distinction between consultant and general practitioner is so well established in Britain that it is widely regarded as an inherent feature of practice. It is therefore remarkable that the roles of the medical workers are very different in different countries at about the same stage of technological development. As a basis for consideration of the organization of medical practice we shall describe three phases in its recent evolution, well illustrated by the services in Australia, Britain and the United States.

The first phase

In the first phase there is no clear distinction between general practitioner and consultant. They are not sharply differentiated by training and appointment, and the practitioner often gives a specialist service.

This was the position everywhere until recently, because medical knowledge did not justify much specialization. The same arrangements may be found in developing countries, where one doctor may have to serve a very large population, and occasionally in thinly populated parts of developed countries, although improved transport should soon make this unnecessary. However this type of practice has also been retained in certain developed countries. In Australia, for example, a considerable amount of major surgery is still performed by general practitioners.

The second phase

In the second phase of practice consultants providing specialized services are clearly identified by training and appointment. The general practitioner selects patients for the consultant who sees only those referred to him. This arrangement is consistent with the complexity of modern medicine but also has disadvantages.

For example, it is possible for specialization to go too far; if all complex services are assigned to consultants, the work which remains may not attract doctors to general practice. There is some evidence that this is the position in Britain today, in criticism of conditions of general practice, and in loss of doctors by emigration. A second disadvantage is the resulting division between hospital and domiciliary services.

The third phase

If the relationship between consultant and general practitioner is uncontrolled, medical practice may enter a third phase. Many doctors prefer to specialize, and when a satisfactory basis for medical practice is not achieved it may fragment into a complex of specialist services. These services are usually based on hospital, and it becomes increasingly difficult to maintain a personal or a domiciliary medical service. This is the situation in some parts of the United States.

Hence none of the three phases of practice exhibited in these countries provides a satisfactory basis for the future relationship between general and consultant practice. In Australia, referral has not gone far enough and services which require specialists are still sometimes in the hands of general practitioners. In Britain, referral has gone too far and the role which remains for the general practitioner is unsatisfactory. In the

United States specialization has gone too far, and it is difficult to maintain personal and domiciliary care.

In the light of these considerations we shall examine the role of the consultant and general practitioner.

THE ROLE OF THE CONSULTANT

The term 'consultant practice' will be used in reference to specialization based on referral of patients. The advance of medical knowledge undoubtedly makes it essential for some doctors to have these conditions for their work, but there are two reasons why they should not be created unless referral as well as specialization is necessary. In the first place, referral to a doctor who can be identified by the patient (for example to an obstetrician by a general practitioner who himself does obstetrics), implies two levels of competence, the patient being asked to go first to the less competent doctor. Accepting that many patients do not need the greater competence, we believe that this is an unsatisfactory arrangement. It is one thing for a doctor to say that he does not do surgery, and quite another to have to admit that although he is responsible for the health of children he is less able than someone else to diagnose and treat most sick children. The second objection to consultant practice if referral is not essential is that the work left to doctors who first see patients may not attract enough graduates to maintain a referral system.

If this interpretation is valid it is not difficult to suggest a basis for consultant practice (specialization based on referral). To work efficiently a neurosurgeon needs both to devote himself exclusively to his field, and the cooperation of other doctors who identify his patients. But no intermediary is needed to tell a pregnant woman that her attendant should be trained in obstetrics, or to inform a mother that her sick child needs the services of a paediatrician. It therefore seems right to limit consultant practice to services involving complex techniques—surgery, anaesthesia, radiotherapy, biochemistry, bacteriology, radiology, etc.—as well as to those of a less technical character where referred work is necessary for expert practice. Perhaps the best example is psychiatry. But consultant practice should not be based on age periods such as childhood or old age, where the patient is able to make his way directly to the appropriate medical attendant. It should be noted that we are saying, not that paediatrics and geriatrics do not require the attention of specialists (we shall later suggest that they do), but only that they should not be based on referred work.

THE ROLE OF THE GENERAL PRACTITIONER

If the consultant is to fulfil the role we have described, the general practitioner must accept responsibility for first contact with the patient, for some services to the patient, and for selection of those who require the work of the consultant. Let us now consider the services which the practitioner should himself provide.

Personal care

The personal role of the general practitioner has been aptly described as follows: 'The doctor we have in mind, then, is no longer a general practitioner, and by no means always a family practitioner. His essential characteristic, surely, is that he is looking after people as people and not as problems. He is what our grandfathers called "my medical attendant" or "my personal physician"; and his function is to meet what is really the primary medical need. A person in difficulties wants in the first place the help of another person on whom he can rely as a friend—someone with knowledge of what is feasible but also with good judgement on what is desirable in the particular circumstances, and an understanding of what the circumstances are. The more complex medicine becomes, the stronger are the reasons why everyone should have a personal doctor who will take continuous responsibility for him, and, knowing how he lives, will keep things in proportion—protecting him, if need be, from the zealous specialist.'

There is widespread support for these views, even where personal medical care is in jeopardy. The reason is not only that most patients prefer to be helped by a doctor they know. It is also that medicine is more than an assembly of specialities, and some doctors should be concerned with the health of individuals rather than with the study of disease or the application of techniques.

Home care

Care at home has long been a feature of medical practice in Britain. Yet some people believe that it is wasteful of the doctor's and the nurse's time. They suggest that the patient should normally go to his doctor's office or clinic, where there are the necessary equipment and assistance. If too ill to do this he should be admitted to hospital.

One objection to this conclusion is economic. If all who cannot go safely to their doctor are to become in-patients, hospitals will be forced to admit many patients with trivial illnesses. Even more serious would be the transfer to hospitals of patients with a considerable degree of disability or infirmity. In countries where the threat of infectious disease has been greatly reduced, the care of the mentally ill and the aged sick is a prominent part of the medical task. It is very desirable that it should be shared with relatives, who with some medical, nursing and social assistance can often make a large contribution to the care of the disabled at home.

Another reason for domiciliary medical care is that it makes it easier for doctors to accept continuous personal responsibility for their patients. Where home care is not provided the tendency is undoubtedly for the service to become impersonal.

Finally it seems desirable for the doctor to be able to influence the patient's domestic environment. Some decisions concerning home arrangements, for example the physical conditions required for the care of an elderly invalid, need to be assessed in the light of medical knowledge. It is very difficult for the doctor to advise on such matters if he never enters the patient's home.

The general practitioner in hospital

One of the most important issues related to the future of medical practice is the role of general practitioners in hospital. In some countries they are able to admit and treat their own patients, and many doctors would regard the practice of medicine as unattractive if they could not. In other countries, including Britain, only a minority of general practitioners enter hospital, where they may serve as clinical assistants without independent responsibility.

There are good reasons why doctors working outside hospital should also have a role inside it. Hospital work provides the best means, perhaps the only means, for a doctor to keep abreast of the rapid advances in medicine which occur during the period of his active work. Moreover the prestige and interest of medicine are now so largely focused on hospitals that most doctors prefer to work in them; and where they are prevented from doing so, the future of medical practice outside hospital, and of personal care, is uncertain.

What work should the general practitioner do in hospital? On the one hand it seems unsatisfactory for him to enter merely for the purpose of maintaining contact with consultants (an arrangement that has been proposed). On the other hand he should not provide services (such as major surgery) for which specialized training and experience are necessary. Whatever the practical difficulties, the aim should be for the general practitioner to perform duties which are compatible with his training, experience and primary responsibility for personal medical care, much of which is outside hospital. It is also desirable that in hospital he should so far as possible continue to serve the patients for whom he is personally responsible at home. The role which most nearly meets these requirements will be referred to after consideration of specialization by general practitioners.

Specialization by general practitioners

Opinion is divided on the question whether general practitioners should specialize. In Britain many doctors consider that family care provides the best basis for their work, and a responsibility for all age groups is scarcely compatible with any significant degree of specialization. But in the United States the work of a doctor is usually restricted, and even in Britain it is by no means uncommon for general practitioners to take a special interest in some field such as obstetrics, paediatrics, geriatric medicine or psychiatry.

While it is impossible to predict confidently the future organization of practice, it should be recognized that it is not easy for a doctor to maintain competence in the care of all age groups. It will become increasingly difficult for him to do so as medical knowledge advances. It is already doubtful whether anyone who gives most of his time to family care can have sufficient experience to deal competently with the occasional unpredictable obstetric emergency. The same is true of geriatrics, where the frequent demands of elderly patients for rehabilitation and prolonged care impose altogether different requirements which may be incompatible with the experience and cast of mind needed in an acute emergency.

If some restriction of responsibility is needed, and this is by no means generally accepted, an attractive basis for it is the age group of the patient. In childhood, in adult life and after retirement the medical problems are relatively homogeneous. Moreover the background of personal and social circumstances is also related to age. For the child, the effects of handicap and illness are largely determined by their influence on his physical and mental development and his education. For the adult they are focused on family responsibilities, particularly reproduction and child care in the case of women, and employment in the case of men. For the individual who has retired, loss of income, occupation and other interests have a considerable bearing on the significance of disease and disability.

It would be consistent with the age pattern of disease and social circumstances to assign responsibility for personal medical care to four classes of doctors: obstetricians, paediatricians, general physicians and geriatric physicians. Each might take continuous responsibility for a defined group of patients, whom he would see usually at the surgery (or office or health centre), but when necessary at home and, we suggest below, in hospital. He would provide both preventive and therapeutic services.

This organization of practice also suggests a possible basis for the work of the personal doctor in hospital. It would be desirable for him to restrict his hospital role to one of the four services with which he was concerned outside. In this way he could often continue to care for his own patients in hospital, transferring them to consultants only for services for which special training and experience are needed. This approach is consistent with the increasing tendency of consultants to restrict their work to a special field of medicine or surgery.

The age-basis is not the only form of specialization in general practice, and many experiments will no doubt be needed to find the best. But we should recognize the limitations of present day arrangements and seek improvements consistent with certain objectives. Among the most important are a personal basis for medical care, provision of some services in patients' homes, a hospital role for the domiciliary doctor and unification of personal preventive and therapeutic services.

SERVICES FOR THE AMBULANT

The site at which the ambulant patient sees his doctor is important for the future of medical practice. In some countries it is usually the doctor's independent office or surgery; but large numbers of patients are also seen at hospital out-patient departments, or at an intermediate facility such as a group practice, health centre or poly-clinic. Before discussing the merits of these different sites we should consider the features which are desirable in the base for services to the ambulant patient.

1. It should be staffed by a number of doctors large enough to make economic use of facilities and ancillary staff. The grouping of doctors in sufficient numbers is also essential to permit some degree of specialization in their work, and to facilitate arrangements for holidays and refresher courses.

2. It should provide facilities for investigation and treatment which would make it possible to do most of the work for the ambulant.

3. It should have an appropriate number of secretaries, nurses, midwives and social workers.

4. It should provide both preventive and therapeutic services.

Judged in the light of these requirements the independent office or surgery is clearly inadequate (although it may be all that is practical in thinly populated areas). It is too small to support enough doctors and ancillary staff or to make economic use of facilities. And although it could conceivably be used for preventive services it is far from ideal for this purpose.

The hospital out-patient department meets, or could be made to meet, all the requirements, and the objections to it are on other grounds. First, it is often too far from the homes of patients, who cannot be expected to go the same distance for preventive services or minor complaints as for investigation or treatment of serious illness. Second, if all ambulant patients are brought to the hospital, it will be burdened with a great deal of trivial illness which will make extravagant use of its resources. And finally, the hospital does not provide the best environment for all medical activities, particularly for those concerned with prevention of disease. For these reasons it seems desirable to restrict the role of the hospital out-patient department to services for which its more elaborate facilities are required.

The third possibility is an intermediate facility of the kind known in Britain as a health centre. It was described admirably in 1942 in the proposals of the British Medical Association's Medical Planning Commission, of which Lord Cohen gave the following account '... The B.M.A.'s model health centre has a different basis. The building and equipment are to be provided by a statutory authority. Medical care for for all insured persons at the centre or in their homes would be provided by G.P.s of the patient's choice. Private patients are envisaged who would attend at the centre or at the G.P.'s private residence or be visited in their own homes. Depending on the size and nature of the area served, and on special needs (e.g. in factories) the centre will house six to twelve practitioners, each of whom will have his own consulting room with a common waiting-room and a small theatre for minor surgery and small X-ray and pathological departments. The centre will have a direct link with a hospital where specialist services (both domiciliary and institutional) would be available and in the hospital might be beds at the disposal of the G.P. for patients whose domestic circumstances are such that, although specialist treatment is not necessary, treatment away from home is desirable. (Some cottage hospitals now offer this type of service.) This scheme also suggests that the centre should assume responsibility for the antenatal, post-natal, infant welfare and school medical services now rendered by the medical staffs of the local authorities. The aims of the centre would be preventive, educational and curative. Each doctor would work at one centre only and each patient would have choice of centre within reasonable geographical limits and would select a doctor from those working at the centre, provided the doctor was prepared to accept him. A unified system of records could be kept and made available at any other health centre in an area through a card index system at a central bureau. The staff would include principals and assistants; the principals to be paid on the basic salary and *per capita* basis from public funds as already discussed, together with private fees. The sale and purchase of practices would cease . . .'

Although written before the National Health Service was introduced this description meets the requirements referred to above. Such a centre would be complementary to the hospital out-patient department, doing the work which, because of its character or relative simplicity, is best kept away from hospital. It would be served by consultants as well as personal doctors, and it would be necessary to send ambulant patients to hospital only when their investigation or treatment needed facilities which would be uneconomic at the health centre.

Centres of approximately this type have been advocated widely in Britain since 1920, and were included among the provisions of the National Health Service. Two main difficulties stood in the way of their construction. One was the reluctance of some practitioners to work in public premises, which were associated in their minds with a salaried service. Their objection is now weaker than in the past and many doctors are willing to work in a health centre. The other difficulty was that the cost of health centres fell on local authorities, who weighed their merits in relation to other expenditure, mainly unrelated to medicine. However the number of health centres has increased in later years, and in time no doubt they will be the main focus of primary and personal medical care.

FURTHER READING

COHEN H. (1943) A comprehensive health service, *Agenda*, **2**, 25.
CARTWRIGHT A. (1967) *Patients and their Doctors*. Routledge and Kegan Paul, London.
FOX, T. F. (1960) The personal doctor and his relation to the hospital, *Lancet*, **i**, 743.
Royal College of General Practitioners (1965) *Present State and Future Needs of General Practice* (2nd Edition). R.C.G.P., London.

22 · PUBLIC MEDICAL SERVICES, 1848–1948

In Chapters 20 and 21 we discussed the evolution of hospitals and medical practice. To complete the account of health services in the period before substantial public responsibility was accepted (in 1848) we should refer briefly to measures concerned with the control of the physical environment.

It is customary to trace the origin of environmental control to the efforts of primitive people to clothe, feed, house and protect themselves. Examples closer to modern practice are to be found in Roman civilization: sewers intended primarily for land drainage, but used also for disposal of waste; wells and aqueducts which supplied water; systems of latrines from which excreta were disposed partly by scavengers in carts, and partly by use of the sewers; and the widespread practice of bathing. But these early measures are distinguished from the control exercised later partly by their objectives, which were social, aesthetic or economic rather than hygienic, and partly by lack of knowledge of their significance to health. They rested on no secure foundation and were largely abandoned in later times.

The earliest measures specifically directed to health were concerned with the isolation of the infectious. From ancient times attempts had been made to segregate lepers, but with this exception it was not until the fourteenth century that even the most rudimentary public health regulations were introduced. They followed the serious epidemic of plague known in England as the Black Death (1348), and were extended in the next three centuries as the disease recurred. Essentially these measures consisted of notification and isolation of infected persons, disposal of infected articles such as clothing (chiefly by burning), and identification and evacuation of the houses of those infected. They were also concerned with the quarantine of individuals who might be suffering from plague, a measure adopted by the City of Ragusa (Dubrovnik) in 1377 and later practised widely elsewhere. Quarantine was first used in London in 1580 to prevent the landing of sailors and goods at the time of an epidemic of plague in Lisbon.

The measures used before the eighteenth century are notable both for their nature and for their limitations. It is surprising that some were of a very practical kind, for ideas about infection and its spread had advanced little from the time of Hippocrates. It is perhaps equally remarkable that once it was recognized that houses and clothing might contribute to the spread of disease, it was not also seen that bad living conditions were everywhere associated with high death rates. Two possible explanations can be suggested. First, attention was fixed primarily on epidemic disease, to which all classes of society were exposed, rather than on the endemic infections which were more conspicuously related to living conditions. And second, the epidemic infections were believed to be due to changes in the atmosphere (referred to as general epidemic constitutions or miasmas) and the control of housing and clothing was considered secondary.

The eighteenth century

During the eighteenth century there was a considerable advance in recognition of the significance of the environment, supported by a demonstration of the effectiveness of its control in prevention of two diseases, scurvy and lead poisoning. The last recorded case of plague in England was in 1669; but in 1719 an outbreak reached Marseilles, and an English physician, Richard Mead, was asked to suggest measures for its prevention. His report, *Short Discourse on Pestilential Contagion*, was widely read. Mead did not reject the prevailing view that infection resulted from corruption of the atmosphere, but he believed that the risk of disease existed only in the immediate neighbourhood of the infected person. These views led him to suggest a far more stringent application of the traditional measures: isolation and quarantine. But he also prescribed much wider changes in the environment—better housing, cleanliness, ventilation, disinfection and control of nuisances—most of which were not adopted until the second half of the nineteenth century.

The significance of the environment was further emphasized by a number of investigations of living conditions. Pringle, an army surgeon, became interested in the relation between bad hygiene in barracks and army hospitals and the spread of infection. He concluded that 'gaol fever', 'hospital fever' and 'ship fever' were the same disease (later identified as typhus) and observed the influence of insanitary conditions on the spread of dysentery. In *Observation on Diseases of the Army* (1752) he recommended improvements in hygiene, diet and clothing, and later attempted to have the same principles applied to civilian hospitals and gaols. A similar series of enquiries and recommendations for the Navy were reported by Lind in an *Essay on the Most Effectual Means of Preserving the Health of Seamen* in 1757, and by Blane in *Observations on the Diseases of Seamen* in 1785.

The examination of association between living conditions and disease was not restricted to the services. It had long been recognized that prisons and hospitals, like ships and army camps, were centres in which and from which infectious diseases spread rapidly. In 1773 Howard, a well-to-do country gentleman influenced by the writings of Pringle and Lind, undertook a Winter's Journey not less poignant than the one that Schubert set to music in the last year of his life. He visited many of the prisons in England, and devoted the remaining years of his life to an intensive study of conditions in prisons at home and abroad. His work showed the association between insanitary conditions and disease, and pointed to the need for reform.

In each of the enquiries to which we have referred the evidence about the association between environment and disease was of an indirect kind. It was essentially the observation that infection and insanitary conditions were commonly found together and did not amount to a demonstration that improvement in any specific feature of the environment resulted in prevention of a specific disease. Many people, including some doctors, remained unconvinced.

Such a position became distinctly less tenable after two experiments in preventive medicine. The first was the demonstration that scurvy could be prevented by eating fresh fruit. This possibility had been suggested at a much earlier date, but it was put beyond reasonable doubt in 1748 by Lind, whose book *Treatise on Scurvy* was largely responsible for the decision that the Royal Navy should provide an adequate supply of lemon juice for ships at sea. The second experiment showed that a form of colic which was endemic in Devon was attributable to lead poisoning. As early as 1739 it had been observed that colic was sometimes associated with cider drinking, but the reason was not clear until 1767 when Baker demonstrated that the illness was caused by the lead in the cider vats and presses.

The nineteenth century

From 1800 the effects of the industrial revolution were much more marked than they had been in the previous century. The new factories required labour, and as many people required work there was a rapid movement of population from the country to the towns. By the mid-century half the population of London had been born outside the town, and in Manchester, Liverpool and Glasgow the proportion was even higher.

One result was a deterioration in working conditions. There was no strong central or local authority with powers to control the location of industries and to impose standards of building practice. Town planning was unheard of, and factories were built without regard for the health of those who had to work in them. Conditions of employment were for all practical purposes uncontrolled. There was no factory inspectorate, no Ministry of Labour and there were few trade unions. If we wish to be reminded that our claim to progressive social policies is of very recent origin, it is only necessary to recall that a hundred and fifty years ago it was possible to exploit paupers; to use female and child labour for much of the underground work in mines; to force a child of 6 to do manual work for 14–15 hours a day for 6 days a week, and to whip him if he faltered; and to expose workers to the risk of industrial disease or accident without obligation to compensate them or their dependants should they fall sick or die.

The domestic environment was also bad. Houses of the poorest type were hastily erected, and are still to be seen in the slum property of industrial towns. In the literature of the nineteenth century there are many descriptions of urban life such as the following by Engels.

'Passing along a rough bank, among stakes and washing lines, one penetrates into this chaos of small one-storied, one-roomed huts, in most of which there is no artificial floor; kitchen, living and sleeping-room all in one ... Everywhere before the doors residue and offal; that any sort of pavement lay underneath could not be seen but only felt, here and there, with the feet. This whole collection of cattlesheds for human beings was surrounded on two sides by houses and a factory, and on the third by the river, and beside the narrow stair up the bank, a narrow doorway alone led out into another almost equally ill-built, ill-kept labyrinth of dwellings ... Everything which here arouses horror and indignation is of recent origin, belongs to the *industrial epoch*. The couple of hundred houses, which belong to Old Manchester have been long since abandoned by their original inhabitants, the industrial epoch alone has crammed into them the swarms of workers whom they now shelter; the industrial epoch alone has built up every spot between these old houses to win a covering for the masses whom it has conjured hither from the agricultural districts and from Ireland.'

The effects of industrialization were superimposed upon hygienic conditions which were already bad. In spite of the advocacy of Mead, Pringle, Lind and others there had been no substantial improvement during the eighteenth century. Methods of supplying water and of disposing of sewage and waste were still primitive, partly because of lack of technical knowledge, and partly because of the absence of public authorities with effective power. Water for drinking purposes was obtained from rivers and streams which were frequently polluted; sewers were open ditches which emptied into rivers; and it was not unusual for householders to dispose of their waste by opening a window and emptying it into the street.

It is scarcely surprising that some people find it hard to believe that mortality did not increase in the early nineteenth century. It is not a matter on which we can be dogmatic, and we have reviewed the evidence, such as it is, in an earlier chapter. We suggested that the undoubted deterioration of the domestic and working environments was counter-balanced by improved nutrition and increased opportunities for employment. The extent of the movement from the country indicates that for many people the choice was between employment in the towns and none at all. Today it is possible to believe that workers are attracted from rural areas by the supposed glamour of town life, but it is hardly credible that any sane person went to industrial areas in the early nineteenth century unless driven by sheer necessity.

THE INTRODUCTION OF ENVIRONMENTAL SERVICES, 1848

At the beginning of the nineteenth century there was virtually no effective public control of water supplies, sewage disposal, housing or foodstuffs. By 1875 all these features of the environment had been subjects of Acts of Parliament. The reasons for introduction of legislation at this time are undoubtedly complex. The period was one of profound social change, of which universal male suffrage (1884) and compulsory education (1870) are notable examples. But some things are believed to have had a special bearing on the pace of legislation concerned with the environment and health.

One was an advance in understanding of the significance of the environment. Even after the demonstrations of Lind, Cook and Baker in the eighteenth century, many people remained unconvinced. This position became almost untenable after the publication in 1842 of a *Report on the Sanitary Conditions of the Labouring Population of Great Britain*. This document, largely the work of Edwin Chadwick, presented the results of an investigation into the relation between environmental conditions and ill-health. By present standards much of the evidence would be regarded as inadequate, but there was a lot of it, and it all pointed in the same direction. Its most significant conclusion was: 'That the primary and most important measures, and at the same time the most practical, and within the recognized province of public administration, are drainage, the removal of all refuse from habitations, streets and roads, and the improvement of the supplies of water.'

Public concern about the environment was also sharpened by experience of infectious disease. Again it was not the prevailing high level of mortality which caused alarm, but the new threat of cholera. This disease, although prevalent in the East, was uncommon in Western Europe and unknown in England before the nineteenth century. It appeared in four major epidemics: 1830–32; 1848–49; 1854; 1865–66. The preventive measures taken were clearly inadequate, and widespread public concern greatly strengthened the hands of those who were pressing the government to act.

We need not trace in detail the history of environmental medicine in the second half of the nineteenth century. The first important measure was the Public Health Act of 1848. Its provisions were essentially permissive, and it was not until the Act of 1875 that some essential features of the environment began to be controlled effectively. These were: water supply; sewage disposal; control of slaughtering of animals; parks and open spaces; isolation hospitals; and a beginning of control of housing. It should be remembered that these changes were introduced with no clear understanding of the nature of infectious disease. Indeed Edwin Chadwick, the most ardent advocate of reform, denied the contagious nature of infection, and throughout his life held the traditional view that it was due to corruption of the atmosphere.

In the same period there was also a notable improvement in circumstances of employment. The first serious attempt at control of working conditions was the Factory Act of 1833, which restricted hours of employment of young children (to 9 hours for children under 9 years, and to 12 hours for children aged 11–18) and introduced factory inspectors. In 1842 Parliament prohibited underground employment of women and girls, and of boys under 10.

The effectiveness of environmental measures was of course greatly strengthened when Pasteur, working first on the nature of fermentation and later on diseases of silkworms, established the bacterial origin of infectious disease. The causal organism of a human disease (anthrax) was first identified by Koch in 1876, and from this time Pasteur, Koch and their followers rapidly laid the foundations of the new science of bacteriology.

In time bacteriology did much more than provide a rational explanation for the success of administrative measures previously taken. It showed how infection is spread, including the unsuspected existence of 'carriers'; it made it possible to diagnose infectious disease with much greater precision; and finally it led to protection against infection by means of immunization.

Although environmental services have improved progressively during the twentieth century, the work of controlling the physical environment is still far from complete. Among the features whose adverse influence on health is still conspicuous in England and Wales are atmospheric pollution, housing, diet, working conditions and road traffic.

The effect of atmospheric pollution is evident in relation to mortality from almost all respiratory diseases, particularly chronic bronchitis and lung cancer. Indeed at the present time in Britain the advantage of rural over urban health, in so far as it is indicated by mortality statistics, appears to be restricted to more favourable experience of respiratory disease. It seems probable, therefore, that the prevention of atmospheric pollution is one of the most important measures now available to health authorities.

The relation of housing to health, although less obvious in national mortality statistics, can scarcely be doubted. There is evidence of the effect of crowding on mental illness and on physical illness, particularly from infectious disease and accidents. Further improvements in housing can therefore be expected to make a significant contribution.

Although gross nutritional deficiency occurs rarely in Britain today, there are two sections of the population whose health may be jeopardized by lack of food. They are old people and the late children of large families. It is among the elderly that need is most common, and in spite of the resources provided by National Insurance and National Assistance their diet sometimes falls below a reasonable minimum. The deficiencies in children are attributable to the fact that the largest families are, in general, the poorest. The late children are exposed to infectious diseases, conveyed by their brothers and sisters, at a time when family resources are at a minimum.

During the present century most of the crude toxic hazards of occupation—mercury, lead, arsenic and phosphorus—have been eliminated or controlled. Nevertheless the standardized mortality ratios indicate that there remain substantial risks associated with employment. Some of them are attributable to low income, but others reflect the effects of the working environment. One of the most obvious adverse features is the industrial atmosphere, which is still responsible for much chronic bronchitis and pneumoconiosis. Another is the high risk of industrial injury. It seems reasonable to believe that in time such risks will be eliminated, but there will remain the possibility that some of the many new organic compounds which are constantly being introduced into industry will prove to be toxic, and constant vigilance will be needed to control them.

The risks to health associated with road traffic are already formidable and are likely to increase. All that need be said about them here is that they will not be reduced without a more radical solution of the traffic problem than any so far applied.

THE INTRODUCTION OF PERSONAL HEALTH SERVICES, 1907

We have reviewed the circumstances which brought a public medical service into existence during the second half of the nineteenth century. By 1900 it comprised local authority environmental and hospital services (for the mentally ill and the infectious) and Poor Law hospital services. The only public provision for patients outside hospital was a limited form of general practitioner service for the destitute. All others had to make and pay for their own arrangements for treatment.

The early years of the twentieth century saw a new phase in the evolution of the public service, the creation of health services concerned with the individual. This had a significant influence on later developments and we must consider the way in which it came about. In broad terms, it resulted from widespread concern about health, particularly of children, and from recognition of the inadequacy of the existing medical services.

By the end of the nineteenth century the improvement in health in England and Wales had been considerable. Mortality had declined continuously for thirty years, and the reduction was large enough to more than offset the effect of a coincident decline of the birth rate on the growth of population. But it was a disturbing feature of the trend that there had been no improvement in mortality in the youngest age group in which the risks of death were still very high. Infant mortality (deaths under one year) was 154 per 1,000 live births in 1900, a good deal lower than in the eighteenth century, but about the same as in 1870. The reason for this is even now not altogether clear. But public opinion was no longer content to accept a high infant death rate as inevitable and had come to believe in the practicability of preventive measures.

Another reason for concern about health was the amount of poverty which remained after more than fifty years of progress. This was demonstrated in two investigations of social conditions, one by Charles Booth in London and the other by Seebohm Rowntree in York. At an earlier period the results might have been dismissed as unrelated to health, but by the end of the nineteenth century the effect of poverty on health was generally admitted, and Simon, the Medical Officer of the Privy Council, referred to it as 'among the worst of sanitary evils'.

Evidence of a more direct kind was provided by the results of inspection of recruits for the Army. In the years 1901–02 40 per cent were unfit for service, the commonest reason being poor physical development, defective vision and heart disease. Reports concerning the health and physical condition of schoolchildren and of adolescents seeking employment in factories were equally disturbing.

An Inter-Departmental Committee on Physical Deterioration dealt widely with public health, and its Report discussed subjects as different as atmospheric pollution, stillbirth registration and the employment of women. It contained two recommendations which were particularly important in relation to the future personal health services: that school-children should be medically inspected at regular intervals; and that school feeding should be undertaken by local authorities.

At this time the only public medical service outside hospitals was the one provided under the Poor Law, which made available to the destitute the part time services of poorly paid general practitioners. Other people had to pay for their medical care, and many did so by voluntary insurance or through friendly societies. It was widely recognized that these arrangements were quite inadequate, and that extension of the public medical service was required. It proved much more difficult to agree about the nature of the extension. Clearly the Poor Law was an unsatisfactory authority to administer medical services, but the kind of organization which should be created was for many years the subject of dispute. Broadly there were two proposals, and the service which eventually emerged was a compromise between them.

The first proposal was that there should be a unified state medical service, based on public health principles, and organized in local areas. This was recommended to the Royal Commission on the Poor Law (1905–09) by the heads of the four Government medical departments, who undoubtedly expressed the views of most doctors in the public service.

The alternative proposal was that the additional public medical services should be provided by doctors in private practice. According to the medico-political committee of the British Medical Association (1909) 'the most satisfactory provision for the treatment of children whose parents cannot afford to pay for it is to place them under the care of private practitioners, who should be adequately remunerated out of public funds independently of the Poor Law'. This was the view of doctors in private practice, and there were indications that at that time many of them would have been prepared to accept a salary for part-time public service.

The full implementation of either of these proposals might have prevented a division between preventive and therapeutic personal services. For the medical staff of progressive public health authorities were then extensively engaged in treatment as well as prevention of disease, and had both been sanctioned by Parliament it can hardly be doubted that a unified service would have grown up, no doubt with serious effects upon private practice. Alternatively, had general practitioners been permitted to undertake the work in schools, and later in child welfare clinics, it is also possible that the division might have been avoided. In this case the attitude of doctors to local authority administration and payment by salary might later have been different from what it was. The Education Act, 1907, and the Maternity and Child Welfare Act, 1918, effected a compromise, by assigning the preventive personal services to public health authorities, while curtailing treatment in deference to the wishes of private doctors.

The School Medical Service, the first personal health service under local authorities, was introduced in 1907. Almost from the beginning it comprised the features which have remained virtually unchanged to the present time: provision of cheap or free food; medical inspections; ascertainment of the handicapped; and treatment. At the outset the treatment of defects discovered in schoolchildren was considered to be a matter for parents to arrange; but it was soon evident that this was quite unsatisfactory, and school clinics were established, mainly for the treatment of minor ailments.

The growth of maternity and child welfare, the second personal health service, was slower than that of the School Medical Service and it was not well established until after the First World War. Until then the service was largely voluntary, and its adequacy varied considerably according to the enterprise and means of local authorities. The Maternity and Child Welfare Act of 1918 established a public service which also has retained its character with remarkably little change until the present time. Its main activities were provision of food, routine inspection, advice to mothers and—in a restricted form—treatment.

NATIONAL HEALTH INSURANCE, 1911

The assignment of personal health services to local authorities, and their restriction essentially to preventive measures, had two important consequences. It made prevention of disease a public responsibility and left treatment as a private one; and it associated the personal health services with environmental medicine and separated them from the services provided by general practitioners and hospitals.

Public responsibility for health services was extended further by the National Health Insurance Act of 1911. Although schemes of this type had existed on the continent of Europe from the late nineteenth century, the Act was a new departure in Britain and was initially resisted by the medical profession. The essential features of the new service were as follows.

(a) It was financed by employer and employee on the insurance principle.

(b) It applied compulsorily to a restricted class of employed persons and did not cover their dependents.

(c) It offered limited benefits—treatment by a general practitioner but not by a consultant or hospital.

(d) It was administered locally by Insurance Committees which were quite separate from the local authorities.

This modest beginning was of considerable significance in the history of health services. It was an extension of public responsibility into therapeutic services, for the first time on a substantial scale. However the responsibility was not assigned to the existing public health authorities under local government, but was placed under a new organization which perpetuated the division between preventive and therapeutic medicine.

THE BACKGROUND OF THE NATIONAL HEALTH SERVICE

Costs of medical care

The most important reason for introduction of a comprehensive health service was undoubtedly the difficulty many people found in paying for treatment. In 1938 the benefits provided under National Health Insurance were available to about 20 million insured workers; rather more than half the population had to meet their own costs or seek assistance from the Poor Law. All hospital treatment had to be paid for according to the means of patients, which were assessed. Many people protected themselves against the risk of hospital expenditure, through voluntary contributory schemes whose rapid growth in the years between the wars reflected the extent of the need.

The combination of public and private finance was unsatisfactory. In principle it was open to anyone in need to appeal to the Poor Law; in practice this safeguard was far from adequate, either because patients were not poor enough to qualify for public assistance, or because they preferred not to be treated rather than apply. The main grounds for criticism of the pre-war medical services were therefore that many patients were inadequately treated, or were placed in financial difficulty by the costs of treatment.

Difficulties of hospitals

Other significant influences were the problems which confronted hospitals. At the outbreak of war rather less than half the hospitals and one-third of the beds were under voluntary bodies; the remainder were under local authorities. (These estimates do not include mental hospitals.) Both systems had their difficulties. Most voluntary hospitals were too small; more than 500 of the 700 general hospitals had less than 100 beds. Many were inadequate in design, staff and equipment; yet because of limited finance it was not possible to remedy the deficiencies. Indeed the voluntary hospitals, originally supported by charitable funds, had become increasingly dependent upon payments made by patients, either directly or through insurance schemes.

The difficulties of the public hospitals were equally serious. They were transferred to local authorities in 1929 at the beginning of a time of extreme financial difficulty, and it was not possible to spend the money required. Inevitably standards varied according to the wealth and initiative of local authorities. Moreover the intention to make hospitals a public health responsibility was far from being realized, and in 1939 almost half the public beds were still administered under the Poor Law. These beds were filled with the mixed population which had long been the responsibility of the Poor Law Authorities, and conditions had not been improved materially by the change in administration.

But the problem of the pre-war hospital service was not merely that there were too few beds and too many unsatisfactory beds. It was also that improvement was prejudiced by the existence of two separate systems of administration.

Uneven distribution of staff

Another difficulty of the pre-war medical services was the uneven distribution of staff between different areas and between different parts of the service. In deciding where to work doctors and nurses are naturally influenced by local circumstances. For personal reasons they choose pleasant places, and for professional reasons they prefer posts where facilities are good. Before 1946 most consultants and nurses favoured general, particularly voluntary, hospitals and general practitioners the wealthier centres. In consequence many public hospitals were inadequately staffed, and there were too few practitioners in the less attractive industrial and rural areas.

It should not be thought that these circumstances which led to a comprehensive health service were peculiar to Britain. How to make medical resources available to everyone is an international problem. Moreover it has recently become more acute, both because modern methods of investigation and treatment have greatly increased the costs of medical care, and because it is now widely accepted that no one should become ill or remain ill for lack of any service which it is possible to provide.

FURTHER READING

Booth C. (1902) *Life and Labour of the People in London.* Macmillan, London.

Engels F. (1892) *The Condition of the Working Class in England in 1844.* George Allen and Unwin Ltd., London.

Rowntree B. S. (1901) *Poverty, a Study of Town Life.* Macmillan, London.

Simon J. (1897) *English Sanitary Institutions* (2nd Edition). Smith, Elder & Co. London.

23 · RELATED SOCIAL SERVICES

Although the risks of epidemic infectious diseases have been shared by all classes of society, it has long been evident that people who are sick are often poor. It has not always been recognized that a considerable proportion of them are sick because they are poor. Until the nineteenth century it was possible to believe that the sick poor were in some way intrinsically inferior, and that an improvement in their circumstances would have little effect on their health, and perhaps only a temporary effect on their poverty. In preferring £5 he would be happy to spend, to £10 he would be unhappy to save, Mr Doolittle in Shaw's *Pygmalion* would have been regarded by some people as typical of a class for which little could be done in respect of health or wealth by public action.

We have seen that the association between poverty and disease began to be recognized during the eighteenth century; but it was not until the publication of Chadwick's *Report on the Condition of the Labouring Classes* in 1842 that the significance of bad living conditions was generally recognized, and not until the identification of bacteria after 1871 that the relationship was understood.

It is understandable that the effect of the environment on health should have been noted first in relation to infectious disease, since it was the threat of infection which led to concern about living conditions. In the present century, however, it has been shown that the effect is by no means so restricted. For example, some nutritional disorders are clearly due to a deficient or ill-balanced diet; and carcinoma of the stomach is an example of a non-infectious illness which is much more common among the poor than among the well-to-do.

In medicine concern with the social services which prevent or relieve poverty is twofold. In the first place, knowing that these services are important to health, doctors have a general interest in their adequacy, and should have something to say about the priority they merit on medical grounds. Secondly, since many patients are ignorant about the services the community provides, some knowledge of them is a desirable part of the equipment of the practising doctor.

The social services will be more intelligible if we consider first the causes of poverty, and the ways in which it can be relieved. The common circumstances in which an individual may require assistance are sickness, disablement (whether temporary or permanent), unemployment, old age, pregnancy, death of a wage earner, inadequate earnings, improvidence and idleness. Although the significance of these causes of poverty has been different at different periods, four have been particularly important: sickness; unemployment; inadequate earnings; and old age.

The methods of financing relief of destitution are charity, voluntary insurance (guilds, sick clubs, commercial insurance), compulsory insurance (financed by employer or employee) and taxation (local or central). In the past assistance was usually from charity and voluntary insurance, but in the present century the trend has been towards increasing reliance on compulsory insurance and taxation.

HISTORY OF SERVICES FOR THE RELIEF OF NEED

The problem which has plagued reformers for as long as there has been public concern with destitution has been to relieve distress without encouraging idleness, to assist an individual when he needs help without diminishing his own efforts to help himself. This dilemma was reflected in the social legislation of three-and-a-half centuries. At some times the paramount consideration was the relief of need, at others the fear of idleness, but the trend has been towards more concern about distress and less about idleness. Nevertheless the problem still exists, although we now prefer to speak of it in terms of security and incentive. The change in terminology is itself significant.

The earliest social services were provided by religious orders, augmented in mediaeval times by the manor houses and by merchant and craft guilds. Many monasteries kept a small hospice or almshouse where poor travellers could get food and temporary shelter, and some provided more permanent care for the sick or weak. In villages feudal lords generally accepted the obligation of caring for their own retainers; in towns merchant and craft guilds practised voluntary mutual aid, while some boroughs provided charities to relieve needy residents of long standing and good character. With the decay of the feudal system and the dissolution of the monasteries many of these social obligations disappeared, and for a considerable period little was done to relieve distress. During the sixteenth century vagrancy and destitution increased so much that it became imperative to deal with them; statutes forbidding vagrancy were common and beggars and wanderers were sometimes beaten or placed in the stocks. By the middle of the century attempts were made to put the poor to work on materials supplied by merchants. Officers of the parishes tried to collect voluntary contributions for the relief of deserving poor, and in a few towns (for example London and Norwich) the principle of a compulsory levy for the relief of the destitute had been accepted.

The Poor Law

Public relief of the poor in England dates from 1601, when the Elizabethan Poor Law Act was passed. It gave to the service a distinctive character which endured for more than three centuries. First, the Poor Law was a local service, administered by unpaid Justices of the Peace and financed by a compulsory parish levy; central direction was weak, and the adequacy of the service varied greatly from one parish to another. Second, the character of the service was in general very harsh; relief was given only in cases of extreme need, and for a considerable period was restricted to residents of long standing. Third, assistance was subject to a test of means of the applicant and his family. The first Poor Law Act stated 'It shall be the duty of the father, grandfather, mother, grandmother, husband, or child of a poor, old, blind, lame, or impotent person or other poor person, not able to work, if possessed of sufficient means, to relieve and maintain that person.' The test of means was very searching, and it had to be shown that both the applicant and his relatives had exhausted their resources.

Throughout the seventeenth and eighteenth centuries the administration of the Poor Law was virtually unchanged. It became somewhat more severe in the early nineteenth century when the economic consequences of the Napoleonic Wars placed a severe strain on its resources. In 1832 a Royal Commission investigated the administration of poor relief, and its report resulted in the introduction of the Poor Law Amendment Act of 1834. Responsibility was transferred from the Justices of the Peace to locally elected Boards of Guardians. The Act attempted to deter applicants, by insuring that relief should not place the recipients in circumstances as favourable as those of the lowest paid labourers, and by requiring recipients to enter an institution. From the early eighteenth century it had been the practice in some areas to make admission to a house of correction or workhouse a condition of assistance. The extension of this practice after 1834 led to the rapid growth of the workhouse system; it also had the unexpected result of establishing an important branch of the hospital service under the Poor Law Authorities.

There was no substantial change in the character of the Poor Law in the late years of the nineteenth century, and at the beginning of the twentieth it was still the instrument of a harsh social policy. Its operation was criticized by the Royal Commission on the Poor Law established in 1905, and a Minority Report of the Commission, largely the work of Sidney and Beatrice Webb, recommended its abolition. In the years that followed other services were introduced which to some extent replaced the Poor Law, or attempted to make up for its deficiencies. It was not until 1948, however, when the National Assistance Act was passed, that the Poor Law was finally abolished.

Workmen's compensation (1897)

For almost three hundred years the Poor Law was the only public service concerned directly or indirectly with the relief of need. The introduction of the Workmen's Compensation Act of 1897 was significant, not only because it introduced the first complementary service, but also because in conception it departed from principles embodied in the Poor Law. Before 1897 it was possible for a worker to obtain compensation for industrial injury or sickness only by proving negligence on the part of his employer; his claim was treated in the same manner as any other claim for negligence, and was not strengthened much by the fact that he was employed. After the 1897 Act the employer was considered to be liable for the results of industrial injury, and it was unnecessary to prove that he had been negligent. In the beginning this principle applied only to specific hazards in a small group of dangerous trades, but in 1906 it was extended to almost every occupation. We should note that the Workmen's Compensation Act provided no public financial or medical assistance to the sick or injured workman; it merely conferred legal rights on him or his dependants, and left them to enforce those rights as best they could by agreement or at law. Even so, the Act was a departure from long established principles in its recognition of some degree of responsibility of an employer for his workers.

Non-contributory Pensions (1908)

A characteristic feature of the Poor Law was its insistence that the recipient of relief should first demonstrate his need. The first departure from this principle was the scheme of old age pensions introduced in 1908. The Old Age Pensions Act provided for a fixed weekly sum to be paid to persons of either sex aged 70 years or more, if they fulfilled certain requirements. These included not only qualifications in respect of nationality and residence, but also the demonstration that the applicant had not failed to work according to his ability, opportunity and need. Once an individual had been accepted, however, the payment was made as of right, and was not subject to the discretion of a public officer. The Act thus made separate provision for an important group of applicants among aged people, and was the first step towards the break-up of the Poor Law.

National Insurance (1911)

The Poor Law and old age pensions were financed by local and central taxation respectively. The National Health Insurance Act of 1911 introduced for the first time in Britain a public service financed in part by insurance contributions. The service included both health insurance and unemployment insurance.

The National Health Insurance Scheme embraced both the limited range of medical services referred to in an earlier chapter, and a weekly sum paid to insured persons who were sick or disabled. Like the medical services, the benefits were restricted to the insured person and in the event of his death were not at first available to his dependants. In 1925, however, an Act of Parliament provided pensions for widows, dependent children and orphans of insured persons, and for insured persons at the age of 65. These new pensions were grafted on to the existing scheme of National Health Insurance.

Unlike health insurance, unemployment insurance in the beginning applied to only a limited section of the working population, to persons in a group of industries with a high level of seasonal unemployment. But the general level of unemployment was so high in the years after the First World War that it was necessary to extend the scope of the Act, and by the mid thirties it included the greater part of the working population. The scheme provided a weekly benefit to be paid for a limited period to eligible unemployed workers.

Like old age pensions, the benefit provided under national insurance was paid as of right, subject only to a record of satisfactory contributions, and to that extent was an improvement upon the Poor Law. Nevertheless there were grounds for serious criticism. In the first place, the level of benefit was not fixed according to basic needs, or adjusted in relation to rising prices. Secondly, it took no account of the size of the family, nor, until 1925, of the needs of dependants after the death of the insured person. And finally, the amount of benefit available in cases of sickness and injury was substantially reduced after a limited period of receipt of benefit.

It will be evident that both the unemployment and health insurance arrangements under the 1911 Act had features which were a distinct advance beyond the provisions of the Poor Law, as well as limitations which made them unacceptable as a final solution of the problem of need.

The Assistance Board

The last major step which preceded the final abolition of the Poor Law was the creation of the Assistance Board in 1934. An Act of Parliament took from the Poor Law responsibility for relief of the unemployed, and transferred it to a new administrative body supported by national funds. The significance of this development can be stated briefly.

In the inter-war years mounting unemployment had made it necessary to extend the scope of unemployment insurance. Even so, many men exhausted their right to insurance benefit, which as we have noted was available only for a limited time, and inevitably turned to the Poor Law for assistance. By this time there had been considerable improvements in the policy and administration of the Poor Law: the workhouse system had been abandoned; scales of relief were more generous than formerly; and in 1929 the basis of local administration had been improved by transfer of the functions of the Boards of Guardians to the Public Assistance Committee of local authorities. Even so, arrangements were still far from satisfactory. Relief was subject to the discretion of the relieving officer and the means test was applied stringently. The incidence of unemployment varied throughout the country and inevitably the demand for unemployment relief often fell most heavily on the poorest local authorities. In 1930 a Royal Commission reviewed the problem of unemployment insurance, and its report was followed by the creation of the Unemployment Assistance Board. It had a dual purpose: to remove from the unemployed the obligation of appealing to the Poor Law and to support the finances of sorely-pressed local authorities. In 1940 it was renamed the Assistance Board, and took from the Poor Law the further task of providing relief for aged persons in need of supplement to their pensions. It later became the principal organ of the central government for making allowances to civilians in financial need because of the war. It was not until 1948, however, that it finally took over the remaining responsibilities of the Poor Law.

THE BEVERIDGE REPORT

In 1941 a committee was appointed by the Government 'to undertake, with special reference to the interrelation of the schemes, a survey of the existing national schemes of social insurance and allied services, including workmen's compensation, and to make recommendations'. The results were published in the Beveridge Report. It was a document of historic importance, not only because it provided a basis for the social legislation which followed, but also because it attempted for the first time to deal compehensively with the problem of poverty.

We have traced the evolution of the public social services concerned with relief of need and have seen that with the exception of the Poor Law they were introduced after the Workmen's Compensation Act of 1897. At the time of preparation of the Beveridge Plan, the main schemes in existence were the Poor Law (1601), workmen's compensation (1897), pensions (1908), sickness and unemployed insurance (1911), and unemployment assistance (1934). The chief criticisms of these arrangements were that they were costly and difficult to administer, and that they left serious deficiencies. The Beveridge Plan aimed to correct these deficiencies.

The Plan was not, however, devised only with regard to existing deficiencies and administrative convenience. It attempted to direct the public social services according to certain principles. One was that relief of need should be only one facet of a social policy concerned with the five giants: Want, Disease, Ignorance, Squalor and Idleness. The other principle was that the social contract between the individual and the state should be based on the idea of security for service. It was intended that the individual should work and contribute when he could, and that when he was unable to work—because of sickness, injury, unemployment, old age or death—the state should provide for him and his dependants. It should be noted that in spite of its humane objectives the Plan had by no means lost sight of incentives. It made service and contribution a condition of benefit; and the scale of benefit was intended to provide no more than the necessities of life. Indeed the Beveridge Report was the first serious attempt to solve on a national scale the age-old problem to which we have referred: to relieve distress without encouraging idleness.

The method suggested in the Report was a compulsory insurance scheme with these features: a flat rate of benefit; a flate rate of contribution; unification of administrative responsibility; adequacy of benefit; all workers, employed and self-employed, to be included.

The crucial feature was adequacy of benefit. The intention was to provide an amount of money, adjusted according to the number in a family, which would be sufficient to meet essential requirements. It was anticipated that the problem of want would thus be dealt with by insurance, and the need for other methods of assistance would be reduced.

PRESENT-DAY HEALTH AND RELATED SOCIAL SERVICES

24 · ORGANIZATION OF HEALTH SERVICES

THE NATIONAL HEALTH SERVICE 1948

In Chapter 22 we discussed the background of the National Health Service (N.H.S.) in the period preceding its introduction in 1948. At that time the health services comprised essentially the following elements: two hospital systems, one voluntary and the other public; personal health and environmental services under local authorities; and general practitioner services financed partly by national health insurance and partly by private payments.

There are several ways in which this organization might have been adapted to meet the needs of a comprehensive service. All three elements might have been brought together under local authorities, and this arrangement was indeed proposed in a White Paper which preceded the Act. However this approach was strongly and effectively resisted by doctors, both general practitioners and consultants, who were opposed to administration of health services by local government. This opposition was undoubtedly influenced by earlier developments, particularly the decisions in 1907 to restrict the personal health services to preventive measures and in 1911 to put National Health Insurance under a separate administration.

It would also have been possible to create a new regional administration for hospitals and consultants and to bring general practitioner services under local authorities. In view of the opposition of doctors in private practice such an approach was not considered seriously. A third possibility would have been to leave the environmental services with local authorities but to transfer their responsibilities for personal health to new local or regional bodies also concerned with general practitioner and hospital services. This was the approach adopted in the revision of 1974, but in 1948 it would have been resisted strongly by local authorities, with their forty years of experience in administering personal health services.

The decisions finally incorporated in the N.H.S. were to leave local authority health services relatively unchanged (except for the transfer of their hospital responsibility) and to create two new and separate administrations, one for general practitioner and the other for hospital (and consultant) services. This meant that while centrally a single government department (the Ministry of Health) was responsible for the N.H.S., locally and regionally responsibility was divided between three authorities, one elected and two appointed. In a little more detail the administration was as follows.

Central administration

The Minister of Health was responsible to Parliament for all the work of the National Health Service. However it should be noted that several other government departments had responsibilities for health activities which remained outside the N.H.S., particularly: the Ministry of Education for the health of school children; the Ministry of Labour for factory hygiene; the Home Office for the care of deprived children and the control of dangerous drugs; the Board of Control for lunacy and mental deficiency; and the Privy Council for medical research. However in the discussion of the N.H.S. and its later revision we shall be concerned only with the responsibilities of the Ministry of Health (later the Department of Health and Social Security).

Hospital and specialist services

The National Health Service Act of 1946 brought all hospital and consultant services under public control and created a new basis for their administration. England and Wales were divided into fourteen Regions, in each of which a Regional Hospital Board (in Wales the Welsh Hospital Board) was made responsible for planning and administering hospital and specialist services, except those in teaching hospitals which were administered separately by Boards of Governors directly responsible to the Minister of Health. In Scotland, where the tradition was different, both teaching and non-teaching hospitals were administered by five Regional Hospital Boards. In Northern Ireland, also, the combined responsibility was assigned to the Northern Ireland Hospitals Authority.

Local authority services

The Act transferred the local authorities' hospitals to Regional Hospital Boards but left environmental and personal health services essentially unchanged. In some respects their responsibilities were extended, for example to include an ambulance service and the care and after-care of certain sick and handicapped persons. The Act also made local authorities responsible for providing, equipping and staffing health centres.

General medical and dental services

General medical and dental services, pharmaceutical services and supplementary ophthalmic services (concerned with sight testing and the supply of spectacles) were administered by Local Executive Councils (L.E.C.s). Their areas were the same as those of local health authorities, but the administrations were quite separate. The chief responsibility of the L.E.C.s was the organization of general practitioner services.

Finance and private practice

The service was financed mainly by taxation and only marginally by insurance contributions. Consultants were remunerated by salary, either full time or part time, according to the number of weekly sessions. General practitioners, who objected to a salaried service, were paid a *per capita* fee for each patient on their lists, and a number of allowances and fees for service.

In this context it should be mentioned that the service allowed doctors to choose their patients and patients to choose their doctors. It also raised few barriers to private practice, except by offering an alternative service which was publicly financed.

THE NATIONAL HEALTH SERVICE IN PERSPECTIVE

It would probably be agreed that the most tangible achievement of the Service was to make medical care available to everyone, and to remove the burden of direct payment from the large number of people who could ill afford it. In addition to this positive achievement it should be said that in the event many of the fears expressed about the public service proved to be groundless. It did not victimize doctors or public; it did not stifle initiative; it did not disturb the relationship between doctor and patient. The limitations were of a subtler kind and were rooted in the tradition of health services.

In retrospect, it can be seen that the National Health Service adopted with only minor changes the framework of services which had evolved in the preceding century. Perhaps the most fundamental weakness of the tradition was that it divided local responsibility. There was no single authority with the duty and power to plan comprehensively, making the best use of resources according to a well-judged scheme of priorities; and the framework of services divided hospital from domiciliary care and preventive from therapeutic medicine. Inevitably there were deficiencies, particularly in the domiciliary and community services and in the care of the elderly, the disabled, the mentally ill and the mentally handicapped. There were also duplications, for example in obstetric and child health services which were divided between local authorities, general practitioners and hospitals.

The consequences of fragmentation were reviewed in 1964 by a national committee which recommended (in the Porritt Report) unification of local health services. This idea was discussed for several years and finally implemented in 1974. The reorganization should be recognized as an event of historic importance, as significant in a different way as the introduction of the N.H.S. in 1948. For it was the first attempt in Britain, and among the first in the world, to recast the framework of services which had evolved, unplanned, in previous centuries.

THE REORGANIZED NATIONAL HEALTH SERVICE IN ENGLAND, 1974

The services brought together in the reorganization of the N.H.S. in England are:

(a) The hospital and specialist services previously administered by the Regional Hospital Boards, Hospital Management Committees and Boards of Governors of Teaching Hospitals.

(b) The family practitioner services, administered by the Executive Councils.

(c) The personal health services, administered by local authorities through their health committees (including ambulance services; epidemiological work; family planning; health centres; health visiting; home nursing and midwifery; maternity and child health care; medical, nursing and supplementary arrangements for the prevention of illness, care and after care; and vaccination and immunization.)

(d) The school health service, administered by the local education authorities.

The N.H.S. is responsible for registration of nursing homes. It is also required to provide school health, child guidance and health education services, but it is recognized that in these cases local authorities are concerned with related activities which require joint planning.

Two very important services continue as responsibilities of local authorities and are therefore outside the N.H.S. These are the personal social services (discussed in Chapter 25) and environmental health, which is interpreted to include: measures for prevention of the spread of communicable disease (other than immunization, some epidemiological investigation and treatment); powers relating to food safety and hygiene, port health and the diseases of animals which affect human health; public health aspects of environmental services; and enforcement of requirements about environmental conditions at work places.

Responsibility for the health of persons in relation to their employment remains with the Department of Employment. The provision of treatment and care of people who suffer injury or ill health through their employment is of course a responsibility of the health authorities.

The framework of the new organization is illustrated in figure 16 and discussed in more detail below.

Central organization

The Secretary of State is responsible to Parliament for national policies related to health and for the administration of the N.H.S. In fulfilling these responsibilities, and assisted by the Department of Health and Social Security (D.H.S.S.), he is concerned with:

1. Establishing national policies and priorities which determine the kind, scale and balance of services to be provided.

2. Agreement with regions and areas on objectives and plans developed in the light of national policies.

3. Allocation of resources to enable regional authorities to put their plans into effect. (It should be noted that family practitioner services are provided separately and are therefore not included in regional and area budgets.)

4. Development of resources essential to the services. This requires specialist work on such matters as personnel (the central Department has special responsibilities in relation to recruitment and training of skilled staff), finance, property and supply.

5. Other functions best organized centrally. They include: certain types of research and preparation of national statistics, purchase of equipment or supplies; supervision of superannuation schemes. The

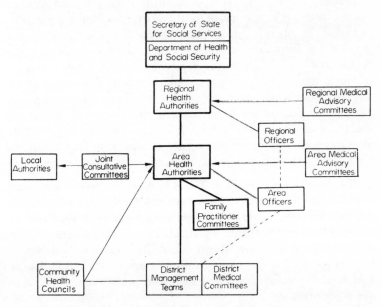

Figure 16. Organization of health services in England.

microbiological service related to communicable disease is administered centrally by the Public Health Laboratory Service Board on behalf of the Secretary of State.

The central Department has some other responsibilities apart from the National Health Service, particularly the personal social services and social security. It is also concerned with licensing of medicines, the control of food safety and hygiene, and acts as the production authority for the medical supply industry.

Regional Health Authorities

Regional Health Authorities (R.H.A.s) are responsible for administration of 14 regions whose boundaries correspond to those of the 14 planning regions formerly used for the hospital service. The Chairman of the R.H.A. and its members are appointed by the Secretary of State after consultation with interested organizations including the universities, the main local authorities and the main health professions. The responsibilities of the R.H.A. comprise three kinds of activity—planning, coordination and supervision and executive functions.

1. *Planning*. The R.H.A. is concerned with strategic plans and priorities derived from a review of needs identified by Area Health Authorities (A.H.A.s); in this role it is guided by national policies. It is also responsible for identification and provision (directly or through the A.H.A.s) of services that need a regional approach, for example, the arrangements for less common specialities such as neurology, neurosurgery, radiotherapy and some types of laboratory investigation. These arrangements affect the deployment of medical, dental and scientific staff. Finally, the R.H.A. has a special responsibility, with the universities, for service facilities needed to support undergraduate and postgraduate medical and dental education, as well as research.

2. *Coordination and supervision*. The R.H.A. has to review area plans, to ensure that they are adequate and attainable, consistent with national and regional policies and coordinated with the work of local authorities. The Regional Authority is particularly concerned where the needs of an area have to be met in part outside its boundaries (for example by a hospital). On the basis of the plans agreed with A.H.A.s, the R.H.A. is responsible for allocating resources and monitoring subsequent performance.

The R.H.A. is also concerned with coordination of services between adjacent A.H.A.s, for example emergency cover, siting and use of ambulance stations and training.

3. *Executive functions.* These include the design and construction of new buildings and works. The more important projects are undertaken directly by the R.H.A.; other building work is delegated to A.H.A.s with regional guidance and approval. Responsibility for operation and maintenance is also delegated to the areas.

4. *Other services.* These include a blood transfusion service and sponsorship of some research projects, for example in epidemiology, requiring regional resources. The region is also responsible for purchase of some —mainly expensive—equipment such as computers, for the computation of statistics and for the provision of selected training facilities.

Regional Officers

The R.H.A. is advised by a Regional Team of Officers (R.T.O.s). They are responsible for advice on such matters as the preparation of a regional development plan, guidelines on priorities and available resources, allocation of resources to areas and reviews of A.H.A.s' performance. However the R.T.O.s are not directly responsible for their counterparts in the area administrations.

Medical Advisory Committees

Reference should be made to the professional advisory mechanism. There are Medical Advisory Committees at both regional and area levels (see figure 16); they are the means of ensuring that in making their decisions both the R.H.A. and the A.H.A. and their staffs take full account of expert opinion.

Area Health Authorities

The revision of the National Health Service followed soon after a re-drawing of local government boundaries and the new health areas were made to correspond with those of local government. There are 72 areas outside London, 38 A.H.A.s corresponding to the non-metropolitan counties and 34 to the metropolitan districts.

The Chairman of the A.H.A. is appointed by the Secretary of State after consultation with the Chairman of the R.H.A. There are approximately 15 members of the A.H.A. appointed by the corresponding local authority, by the University (areas with substantial teaching facilities are administered by 'teaching' A.H.A.s) and by the R.H.A. after consultation with the main health professions and other organizations. While the A.H.A. always includes professional members their number is not prescribed.

The functions of the Area Authority comprise both planning and operation of services.

1. *Area planning*. In cooperation with the R.H.A. and corresponding local authority, the A.H.A. is responsible for the planning and development of services designed to meet the national and regional objectives. This requires appraisal of existing services and identification of their deficiencies.

2. *Area operation of services*. Although the day-to-day running of services is based on the districts, the areas have certain operational responsibilities. The A.H.A. is the employer of staff who work at area headquarters and in the districts. It is also responsible for supporting services such as catering and domestic work.

Area Officers

Like the R.H.A., the A.H.A. is advised by a team of officers whose role, with some differences, is analogous to that of their opposite numbers working in the regional authority. Their responsibilities include: assistance to districts in their planning and review of district plans and budgets; preparation of matching plans jointly with local authorities; monitoring and coordination of the work of the districts; responsibility for certain area services. Finally it should be noted that area officers do not manage their district counterparts, both area and district staffs being directly accountable to the A.H.A.

Local Joint Consultative Committees

There is a considerable overlap in the interests of health and local authorities, for example in relation to education, environmental health, housing, personal health and social services. The position is complicated by the fact that the local government services in such fields are not all administered by the same authorities. In the revision of the N.H.S. it was therefore essential to seek ways, in addition to common boundaries, in which collaboration between health and local authorities could be ensured.

One of these was by introduction of Local Joint Consultative Committees. They are composed of members of the two authorities, and their function is to advise on the planning and operation of services in spheres of common interest.

Family Practitioner Services

The reorganization of health services did not change the status of general medical and dental practitioners, ophthalmic medical practitioners, opticians and pharmacists; all of them continue, as before, to provide services as independent contractors. So while it was hoped that general practitioners would develop and, in some cases modify their work to make it an integral part of a comprehensive service, the Area and Regional Authorities have no responsibility or power to bring this about.

The A.H.A. is responsible however for developments where general practitioner services involve other parts of the service. These include planning and development of health centres, plans for contractor services in new towns or redevelopment areas and arrangements for nurses and other skilled staff employed by the A.H.A. to work with general practitioners. The A.H.A. in turn has to ensure that its plans affecting contractor services are acceptable to general practitioners.

Family Practitioner Committee

The contracts involving general practitioners are administered by a Family Practitioner Committee set up by the A.H.A. It is responsible for contracts with practitioners, administration of terms of service (including remuneration schemes) and statutory disciplinary arrangements. The composition of the Committees is similar to that of the L.E.C.s which they replaced: half the members are professionals appointed by the local professional committees and the remainder are appointed by the A.H.A. and local authority.

In the light of these arrangements we may summarize the relation of the administration of the National Health Service to the doctors providing clinical services. In hospital (including consultant) and personal health services the doctor's day-to-day work is a matter for his own judgement but the administration is responsible for the services provided. In the case of general practitioner services, however, Regional and Area authorities have no direct responsibility, except in relation to those parts of the work of the general practitioner which impinge on other services.

District Administration

The day-to-day running of the National Health Service is based on districts. Their size and number was determined by the size of population considered suitable for administration of local health services, usually between 150,000 and 250,000. Each district was planned to contain a district general hospital.

It is important to emphasize that the district is not a separate level of administrative authority, analogous to area and region. Rather it is a part of the area administration, so organized as to enable the A.H.A. to meet community needs most effectively. The district administration includes the District Management Team and District Medical Committees.

The District Management Team (D.M.T.)

The D.M.T. consists of a consultant, a general practitioner, the District Community Physician, the District Nursing Officer, the District Finance Officer and the District Administrator. These officers are all jointly and equally responsible for district management. Their responsibilities are essentially to administer most of the services of the N.H.S. at district level. They are expected to assess existing services and to propose improvements which are possible within the resources available. Their proposals are discussed with the area officers, and finally submitted to the A.H.A. for approval and financial support.

The District Medical Committees (D.M.C.)

In each district there is a D.M.C. which represents all general practitioners and specialist staff (including dentists) working in the district. Its role is to coordinate the medical aspects of health care throughout the district and in this work it is expected to cooperate with the D.M.T. This mechanism is intended to ensure that developments at district level reflect the views, and in general have the support, of all medical and dental practitioners.

The Specialist in Community Medicine: The District Community Physician

In the reorganization of the N.H.S. the term 'specialists in community medicine' was introduced to describe medically qualified administrators, most of whom were employed formerly by local health authorities (medical officers of health) and at Regional Hospital Boards. However their role has been modified considerably in the reorganized service and they now work in posts at regional, area and district level.

The specialist in community medicine has three main functions. First, as a specialist he is expected to provide information for clinicians and to advise on alternative approaches to care, having particular regard for the relation between health and local authority services. Second, as a manager, he is concerned with planning of services, with provision and interpretation of information, with evaluation of services and with preventive measures and the deployment of clinical doctors in public health (for example in relation to immunization, screening, health education and chiropody). Third, he has a special role in relation to local authorities, particularly in respect of advice and services in three areas: environmental health, child health including school health, and personal social services.

The District Community Physician has already been referred to as a member of the district management team. Here his role is to identify opportunities to improve the health care services, to coordinate the work of health care planning teams, to coordinate the preventive services in the district and to advise his consultant and general practitioner colleagues on matters falling within the scope of community medicine. In some areas (not all) he also advises the local authority on environmental health and has responsibilities in relation to the school health service.

Community Health Councils

One of the most important issues raised by the organization of health services is the role of the public in their evolution and administration. At the beginning of this chapter it was noted that in its original form the N.H.S. left personal health services with local authorities but created separate administrations for hospital and general practitioner services. In unifying the services, the 1974 revision transferred the personal health services to the new regional, area and district administrations described above. This finally took from local authorities responsibility for personal health care, with which they had been associated in various ways for about a hundred years. There are many critics of this decision, particularly among those who consider that health services should be administered by the elected local authorities who are directly accountable to the public who provide the finance.

In the reorganized service the views of the consumer are represented by the Community Health Councils. There is one Council for each district and its role is to represent to the A.H.A. the interests of the public. In order to do this it has power to secure information about the services, to visit hospitals and other institutions, and to have access to the A.H.A. and its officers. The A.H.A. in turn is expected to consult the Councils about developments, particularly those (such as closure of hospitals or change of use of facilities) in which the public is likely to be particularly concerned. Apart from such lines of communication and influence, the Councils have no direct responsibility for the planning and administration of services.

Finance

The financial structure of the reorganized services is essentially the same as that of the original N.H.S.: the costs are still met mainly from taxation, from moneys voted by Parliament for health services. The D.H.S.S. makes capital and revenue allocations to the R.H.A.s which in turn allocate funds to A.H.A.s. Payments to general medical practitioners, it is important to note, are funded separately by the Department and not through the R.H.A.s. The new N.H.S. also recognizes the special financial needs of 'teaching areas', that is for those which have substantial facilities used for medical and dental education and research. The R.H.A. receives from the Department a specific identified allowance for teaching and research and it is the responsibility of the R.H.A. to use these funds to ensure that facilities related to teaching and research are adequate in the 'teaching areas'.

Perhaps the chief variation in the earlier financial arrangements was the relief to local authority expenditure which resulted from the transfer of responsibility for their personal health services to the new unified administration.

Arrangements for London

It was necessary to make special arrangements for London, where there were features affecting the planning and administration of health services. Among these features were the established pattern of local government, the types and distribution of hospitals (with a large number of separate undergraduate and postgraduate teaching hospitals) and the fact that general practitioner services were administered over areas much wider than the individual London boroughs. In the new organization the borough boundaries are used in forming health A.H.A.s although some services (for example general practitioner and ambulance services) still use wider boundaries.

In London there are four R.H.A.s, each of which inevitably contains teaching areas. The A.H.A.s comprise single boroughs or groups of boroughs, but the health districts do not always conform to borough boundaries. The ambulance service continues, as formerly, to be administered as a single service for the whole of Greater London. The planning of teaching hospitals, particularly postgraduate hospitals, presents particular problems in London and although postgraduate hospitals are intended to come ultimately into the usual framework, for an interim period they continue to be administered by Boards of Governors financed directly from the D.H.S.S.

THE ORGANIZATION OF HEALTH SERVICES IN OTHER PARTS OF THE UNITED KINGDOM

In general, the aims of the unification of health services in 1974 were common to all parts of the United Kingdom. Nevertheless there is some variation in the pattern of administration, determined both by the tradition of services in each country, and by the smaller size of the populations which required some modification of the organization described for England. In Northern Ireland there is the important difference that health and social services are administered by the same authority.

Wales

Although the administrative structure of the health service in Wales is similar to that in England, it differs in a number of respects.

It was considered unnecessary in a country with less than three million inhabitants to interpose a regional health authority between the A.H.A.s and the Welsh Office (the central government department). Consequently there is no R.H.A. and the Welsh Office is responsible for strategic planning within the Principality and for monitoring the performance of the eight A.H.A.s. Professional advice is available to the Secretary of State for Wales from committees representative of the main health professions in Wales and from the Welsh Council, as well as from bodies advisory to the Secretary of State for Social Services.

In all main areas of planning and decision making there is a substantial delegation of responsibility to A.H.A.s. But a special body— the Welsh Health Technical Services Organization—is responsible for certain specialized and technical supporting tasks. These include the design and execution of major capital works, the systematic evaluation of contracting arrangements for supplies, and a computer-based central management information service.

As in England, the boundaries of the A.H.A.s are coterminous with those of the local authorities. Consequently the A.H.A.s in Wales serve much smaller populations; indeed at least three of them have smaller populations than would be considered appropriate for a district in England and the population of one (Powys) is so small and scattered that it has no district general hospital within its boundaries.

Scotland (figure 17)

Health services in Scotland were reorganized under the National Health Service (Scotland) Act, 1972. The principles behind the reorganization were essentially the same as in England but there are some differences in the administration of the services.

Central administration

The health services are the responsibility of the Secretary of State for Scotland working with the Scottish Home and Health Department. The Department is advised by a Health Services Planning Council, with members appointed by each health board (see below), by each university with a medical school and by the Secretary of State for Scotland. The Planning Council in turn is advised by National Medical Consultative Committees. There is also a Common Services Agency whose function is to provide the Departments and Health Boards with a variety of executive and advisory services which are necessary throughout Scotland and can be provided most efficiently by a single agency. Examples of the Agency's work are the planning and execution of major building projects and central functions in relation to research and intelligence and health education.

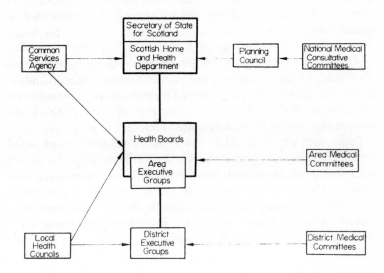

Figure 17. Organization of health services in Scotland.

Area administration

Scotland is divided into 15 areas each of which is the responsibility of a Health Board. The population served by Boards varies, from 1,700,000 in Glasgow to below 100,000 in some parts of the mainland and on the Islands. Boards are directly responsible to the Central administration, which provides the finance for the development and maintenance of an integrated health service. In Scotland the Health Board is the authority with which general practitioners have a contractual relationship. The senior officers of the Health Board function as an Area Executive Group and the Board is advised by Area Medical Committees. In areas which include a medical school there is provision for a University Liaison Committee.

District administration

Except in very small areas there is a subordinate management structure, the majority of areas being divided into two or more districts. Districts are concerned with the operation of the service rather than with the major decisions on planning and policy which are matters for health boards and the central administration. The senior officers of the district operate as an Executive Group and are advised by District Medical Committees.

Every Health Board is required to establish a Local Health Council or Councils for their area or for districts within the area. The role of the Councils is analogous to that of the Community Health Councils in England; that is to say, they have no executive powers, but represent the interests of the public by assessing the adequacy of the health services provided in the area or district.

Differences which should be noted in the organization of health services in Scotland (compared with England) are: (a) the responsibilities of the Regional and Area Health Boards (England) are combined in the Health Boards and (b) general practitioner services are, financed and administered by the Health Boards rather than by a separate body (the Family Practitioner Committee) which receives its finance directly from the central Department.

Northern Ireland (figure 18)

In Northern Ireland major policy decisions are made by the Ministry of Health and Social Services of Northern Ireland under The Health and Personal Social Services (Northern Ireland) Order 1972. The services are administered within this policy by four Area Boards covering the Eastern, Northern, Western and Southern areas of the province. These areas are bounded by local government district boundaries and include several districts in each area. Within an area local government districts are linked for the purpose of the management and delivery of health and personal social services. These conjoined local government districts are called Health and Personal Social Services Districts.

Members of the Area Board are appointed by the Minister. Some are nominated by the Local Government District Councils; others are professional people such as doctors, nurses and social workers, appointed after consultation with the professional organizations; and the remainder include businessmen, trade unionists, and members chosen from the universities and colleges and voluntary organizations dealing with health and social problems.

Each Area Board is served by four main committees; a Health

Services Committee, a Social Services Committee, a Policy and Resources Committee and an Administrative Services Committee.

Most of the work of the Boards is delegated to professional officers, who constitute the Area Executive Team. This consists of a Chief Administrative Officer, a Chief Administrative Medical Officer, a Chief Administrative Nursing Officer, the Director of Social Services and the Chairman of the Area Medical Advisory Committee. The later committee represents all the specialities and general practice in the area.

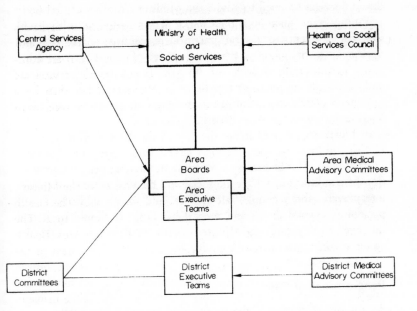

Figure 18. Organization of health services in Northern Ireland.

At the level of the Health and Personal Social Services Districts there is also an Executive Team composed of five District Officers corresponding to the chief Area Officers. This district team is responsible for the delivery of health and personal social services to the individual. It is advised by a District Medical Advisory Committee composed of representatives of specialists and general practitioners in the district.

An important innovation in the new health service is the creation of District Committees which are intended to represent 'consumer' interests. These Committees are appointed by the Area Board and members include local government councillors and representatives of local voluntary organizations. They have no executive power but have the right to visit hospitals, hostels, and homes for children and the elderly to assess the quality of the services provided and make recommendations.

There are a number of central advisory committees whose chairmen, along with the chairmen of the Area Boards, constitute a Health and Social Services Council to advise the Minister. Another central body with important functions is the Central Services Agency. It is responsible for payments to general practitioners, dentists, pharmacists and opticians; for the selection and appointment of consultants and other senior hospital staff on behalf of the Area Boards; for legal services; and for central contracts for supplies.

General practitioners continue as independent contractors and their contracts are with the Area Boards.

In Northern Ireland, unlike the rest of the United Kingdom, the Health and Personal Social Services have been integrated at Area and District level. This had many advantages in the treatment and prevention of conditions in which the social and medical aspects are closely interwoven, for example, alcoholism and other addictions, self poisoning, mental illness and mental handicap. It should be noted, however, that centrally the Ministry of Home Affairs is responsible for children taken into care and for adoption.

Programmes of Care

An important change in the reorganized service is the setting up of Programmes of Care to tackle specific problems such as those mentioned in the preceding paragraph. The Area Executive Team, having decided that a certain problem might benefit from this approach, sets up a planning team of experts and others. For example, if the problem were mental handicap the team might include a psychiatrist working in the field of mental handicap, a psychologist, a social worker, an administrator, a general practitioner, an epidemiologist, an educationist and a representative of the voluntary organization concerned with the welfare of handicapped children. This team would then study the size and nature of the problem in their area, the existing facilities for care, treatment and prevention and would identify deficiencies. Finally they would make recommendations for the improvement of the health and personal social services for the mentally handicapped, which would be implemented, if agreed, by the Area Board.

25 · ORGANIZATION OF RELATED SOCIAL SERVICES

POST WAR SOCIAL SERVICES

Relief of Need

The discussion of the evolution of social services related to health in Chapter 23 was focussed on services directed to the relief of need. Beveridge had recommended that these services should be financed in future mainly by insurance, and he anticipated that if the levels of benefit were adequate there would be less need than formerly for public assistance of other kinds. Parliament attempted to implement these proposals by passing four Acts: The National Insurance Act, 1946; the National Insurance (Industrial Injuries) Act, 1946; the National Assistance Act, 1948; and the Family Allowances Act, 1945. The first three were concerned with insurance and assistance, and the fourth made provision for payments to families according to the number of children. The object of the last was to relieve the burden in large families where the stress of poverty and ill-health was sometimes severe.

In one important respect post war developments departed from Beveridge's proposals: the levels of benefit paid under national insurance were never adequate and it was therefore necessary to rely heavily on assistance. The reason for this was largely outside the control of the government; it was due mainly to the rise in the post war cost of living and, to a lesser extent, to the granting of retirement benefit to persons who had contributed for only a short period. The inflation, and the resultant difficulties, have continued to the present day, so that there is still the imbalance between insurance and assistance which Beveridge hoped to avoid.

Other social services

Other public social services originated in the Poor Law, which, under its general responsibilities for the destitute, made provision for, *inter alia*, orphaned and deprived children, the mentally ill, the mentally subnormal and the aged poor. However, with the break up of the Poor Law these responsibilities were transferred to other departments of the local authority and the process was completed in 1948. In that year the Children's Act required local authorities to appoint a Children's Officer and to establish a Children's Committee with the duty of caring for deprived children. A later Act extended these obligations and provided the basis for preventive action which would 'promote the welfare of children by diminishing the need to receive children into or keep them in care'. The National Assistance Act, 1948, by taking from the Poor Law responsibility for financial assistance to those in need, provided the basis for the welfare services of local authorities, which included accommodation and other services for the elderly, the physically handicapped and the homeless.

Another group of personal social services developed under local authorities in association with their health services. As early as 1918 the Maternity and Child Welfare Act empowered local authorities to employ home helps for mothers in the lying-in period and during the Second World War this service was extended to other classes such as the sick and infirm. Local authorities had acquired responsibilities for the mentally ill and mentally subnormal and these were increased considerably in the post war period. Their duties under the National Health Service to prevent illness and provide care and after care also involved them in extensive social services, particularly in relation to the infectious, the chronic sick and problem families.

Yet another class of local authority social services evolved in conjunction with education, for example enforcement of school attendance, special educational facilities for handicapped pupils, provision of free meals and child guidance. Finally we should refer to the considerable welfare functions developed by housing departments in their work on slum clearance, redevelopment and rehousing.

THE SEEBOHM COMMITTEE

The local authority and allied personal social services were reviewed by a government committee which published its recommendations in 1968. At that time the services were divided between the children's, welfare, health, education and housing departments of local authorities. The Committee concluded that the services were deficient in quality and quantity, and as examples they cited the waiting lists for day and residential care for the mentally ill, the mentally subnormal, the handicapped and the aged. The services were also thought to be poorly coordinated and difficult of access by the public. The Committee attributed these deficiencies mainly to lack of resources and to the division of responsibility for the social services between several departments of local authorities.

The solution for these difficulties suggested by the Seebohm Committee was unification of the social services in a comprehensive social services department. The services proposed for inclusion were:

(a) the services provided by children's departments;

(b) the welfare services provided under the National Assistance Act, 1948;

(c) educational welfare and child guidance services;

(d) the home help service, mental health social work services, other social work services and day nurseries, provided by local health departments;

(e) certain social welfare work undertaken by some housing departments.

THE REORGANIZED SOCIAL SERVICES

The social services were reorganized under the Local Authority Social Services Act, 1970, which gave effect to three of the recommendations listed above—(a), (b) and (d). (The Act made no reference to the welfare services provided by the education and housing departments, as these are not statutory services and no legislation was necessary. In the case of the child guidance service, so many agencies—health, education and children's—were concerned, that it was felt that any legislation would be unnecessarily complicated.) Local authorities were required to unify the services under a Social Services Committee and to appoint a Director with responsibility for administration of the following services.

Services for children and mothers

In general the services are responsible for promotion of the welfare of children and in some cases, mothers. The work includes responsibility for children who cannot be cared for in their own homes and are said to be 'taken into care' (orphans, deserted children, some children suffering from mental disorder, etc.); arrangements for adoption; protection and care of the young in relation to criminal proceedings; provision of day care of children under 5 years, including day nurseries and child minding; care (including residential care) of unsupported mothers.

Services for old people

These are services concerned mainly with the provision of care for older people, either in the community or in residential establishments. They include the home help service, meals on wheels and old people's homes. They are also concerned with protection of property when people are removed to hospital and with defraying of funeral expenses of those who die with no finances to cover the cost of burial.

Services for mentally ill and mentally subnormal people

The services promote the welfare of persons suffering from mental disorder (mental illness or mental subnormality), for example by providing residential accommodation and making arrangements for training and employment. They include responsibility for the welfare of the mentally disordered in hospital.

Services for physically handicapped people

The services are concerned with the welfare of persons who are blind, deaf, dumb or otherwise physically handicapped. They include provision of facilities for training and employment of the disabled.

The reorganization of health and social services described in this and the preceding chapter has separated the administrations of the two services in the United Kingdom, except in Northern Ireland where they are under the same authority. Social services have been unified under local authorities; health services, including personal health services, have been placed under a new and separate administration. In Chapter 24, we considered the reasons, largely rooted in history, why health services were not placed under local authorities. The Seebohm Committee, after reviewing various alternatives, came to the conclusion that it was desirable to create a comprehensive social service department under local government.

The grounds which influenced the Seebohm Committee in this decision did not persuade all medical people. Some were particularly concerned about the separation of responsibility for health and welfare of the elderly and physically handicapped, whose medical and social needs are intimately related, if not inseparable. There was criticism of the decision to separate from health services the social services for the mentally ill and mentally subnormal, whose social and medical needs are also closely associated. However the Committee concluded that these objections were outweighed by the advantages which would result from a unified social services department, and this conclusion was accepted in the reorganization of the services.

26 · OBSTETRIC SERVICES

The health needs of a pregnant woman can be stated simply. First, she should have a medical examination early in pregnancy to ensure that her general health is good, and another some time after delivery to determine whether it has been in any way impaired. Second, at regular intervals during pregnancy, labour and the puerperium she requires the help and advice of a skilled attendant. And third, at any stage, she should have immediate access to specialist hospital services if the need arises.

But although these requirements are easily summarized it is by no means obvious how they are best met. Organized obstetric services are of comparatively recent origin and they are still not entirely satisfactory. It will be easier to understand their present organization if we consider first the way in which they have evolved.

EVOLUTION OF SERVICES

Until the nineteenth century midwifery was almost exclusively a woman's province. From that time an increasing proportion of women who could afford to do so paid a doctor to attend them, but the large majority continued to be delivered by midwives. No control was exercised over their activities; they had no recognized training, no representative organization, and except in the case of the few hospital-trained midwives their standard of practice was very low. Charles Dickens's Sairey Gamp was the prototype, with her request for refreshment 'to be brought regular and draw'd mild'. The foundation of the Midwives' Institute (1881) and the passing of the first Midwives' Act (1902) marked the beginning of standardized training and regulated practice.

Except for the few who worked on the district from teaching hospitals, all midwives earned their living by private practice. The rapid extension of hospital midwifery and the decline of the birth rate put many out of business, and after the introduction of a wholetime salaried municipal midwife service in 1936, few private midwives remained. From this time domiciliary midwifery became for all practical purposes a local authority monopoly.

Hospital obstetrics

The founding of the Rotunda Hospital in Dublin in 1745 and the establishment of a few lying-in beds in London teaching hospitals mark the beginning of medical interest in obstetrics. But for the next 150 years the growth of hospital maternity services was slow compared with the remarkable expansion of other hospital facilities. The reason is not far to seek: the maternal death rate in lying-in hospitals was so high that few women chose to be confined there. In the Maternité of Paris, for example, maternal mortality between 1861 and 1864 was 124 per 1,000 births. This is hardly surprising when it is remembered that midwife pupils attended normal labours and fever cases alike, and doctors often went to women in labour from postmortem room and surgery without removing their top-hats and frock-coats or washing their hands.

By the end of the nineteenth century, it became clear that puerperal fever was often spread by doctor and midwife and could be prevented by cleanliness and routine disinfection of the hands. At the same time anaesthesia and antiseptic techniques were making obstetrical interference less disastrous. For the first time mortality rates in hospitals began to bear comparison with those at home. The proportion of confinements in hospital has continued to increase. It was 30 per cent in the nineteen twenties, 60 per cent in the nineteen fifties and is now approaching 90 per cent.

General practitioner obstetrics

Although medical obstetric specialists were well established in most large towns by the beginning of the nineteenth century, the practice of midwifery by doctors was still frowned upon by the Royal Colleges. In 1827 the President of the Royal College of Physicians wrote to Sir Robert Peel that the practice of midwifery was 'an act foreign to the habits of gentlemen of enlarged academic education'. There was, however, an increasing demand from well-to-do women for doctors to attend them, and in 1868 the General Medical Council insisted that medical students must conduct 20 labours before sitting their final examination. Since the Medical Act of 1886 qualification in midwifery as well as in surgery and medicine has been required for registration.

A considerable barrier to an efficient midwifery service was the cost of medical care. The National Health Insurance Act of 1911 made no provision for maternity, other than the payment of a small cash benefit to the woman insured in her own right. In 1918 the principle of fees paid from the public funds (recovered if possible from the patient) to medical practitioners called in by midwives in emergencies was accepted. Within the National Health Service there are now no financial barriers.

Antenatal clinics

The need for regular antenatal supervision is today a commonplace, but fifty years ago it was unheard of. As hospital practice expanded, antenatal clinics slowly became an accepted feature of hospitals with lying-in beds. They served partly as supervisory centres for booked cases and partly as clinics to which outside doctors could send cases for a consultant opinion. At the same time local authorities began to set up voluntary supervisory centres, staffed by their own doctors. The two services developed side by side, but made little contact with one another.

Obstetric services before the National Health Service

The diverse origins of the obstetric services explain their complicated pattern before the introduction of the National Health Service. About half the confinements in England and Wales were in voluntary or municipal hospitals, but criteria for hospital admission were not at all clearly defined. The hospital usually accepted responsibility for antenatal supervision of its booked cases, but occasionally part of the supervision was provided by the patient's general practitioner or the district antenatal clinic.

The other half of the confinements were at home, attended by municipal midwives. The midwife accepted responsibility for antenatal care, working in close cooperation with local authority doctors and health visitors at the district antenatal clinic. These women were referred to hospital or to their own general practitioner should the clinic doctor discover any contraindication to domiciliary delivery during the antenatal period. If difficulty arose during labour or the puerperium, a local general practitioner was called and his fee paid by the local authority according to a scale fixed by the Ministry of Health.

A small proportion of women arranged for their general practitioner to attend them at home or in a private nursing home. In such cases a municipal or private midwife assisted the doctor. He accepted responsibility for antenatal supervision, but sometimes the woman also attended a local authority clinic. If an emergency arose during confinement, a consultant obstetrician was called in.

Obstetric services under the National Health Service

The introduction of National Health Service effected two immediate changes in obstetric services: local authorities lost their maternity hospitals to Regional Hospital Boards and women became entitled without charge to a maternity medical service if they decided to have their babies at home. There were also two important long-term effects: local authorities are no longer concerned with antenatal care or domiciliary midwifery and hospital delivery, often in a short-stay unit, has become the accepted norm. Women booked for hospital delivery receive a first comprehensive antenatal examination at the hospital and then, if there are no abnormalities, their general practitioners provide antenatal care until about the thirtysecond week. From then until delivery they attend the hospital antenatal clinic. A small proportion of women elect to receive their antenatal care from general practitioner obstetricians and are delivered in general practitioner maternity units.

Two other important developments should be mentioned: the changing attitude towards abortion and the growth of family planning and birth control services. The Abortion Act (1967) introduced legal abortion into the United Kingdom, with the provision that two doctors must agree that the mental or physical health of the mothers of children would be seriously affected by the birth of the child. Under the National Health Service (Family Planning) Act, 1967, local authorities were given power to provide contraceptive advice for women on medical or social grounds, and in 1974 contraceptives were made available on prescription as a regular part of the Health Service.

APPRAISAL OF OBSTETRIC SERVICES

Achievement

From contemporary records of hospital and private practice, and from what is known of maternal mortality in underdeveloped countries today, it seems probable that 150 years ago at least 10 women died in

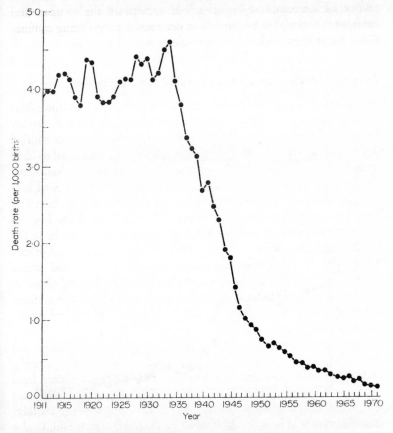

Figure 19. Maternal mortality rate England and Wales 1911–1971.

childbirth for every 1,000 births. When puerperal fever assumed epidemic proportions mortality sometimes increased tenfold. By the end of the nineteenth century the level had fallen to below 5 per 1,000 in England and Wales, but from that time it did not decline much until the mid-thirties. The rate then fell rapidly, and it is now less than 0·2 per 1,000 total births (figure 19).

The reason for the trend of maternal mortality in the nineteenth and early part of the twentieth centuries is not clear. The decline since 1935 can be attributed first to the control of sepsis by chemotherapy and antibiotics, second to the control of haemorrhage associated with the introduction of a national blood transfusion service and third to a fall in mortality from toxaemia, partly explained by improved nutrition and better antenatal care (figure 20). However, although a great deal has been achieved, confidential enquiries into maternal deaths indicate that even at their present low level about half of them are associated

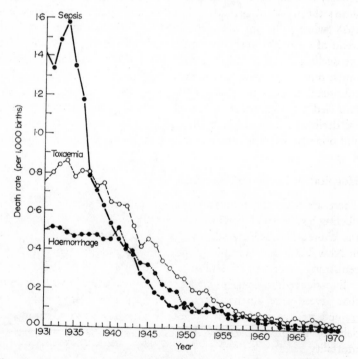

Figure 20. Maternal mortality rates due to sepsis, toxaemia and haemorrhage. England and Wales 1930–1971.

with an 'avoidable factor'. This does not necessarily mean that in all these cases death could have been prevented. But it does imply that some aspect of the mother's care fell short of what should be expected from a comprehensive obstetric service. For example haemorrhage is an important cause of death—which is largely preventable—and deaths from toxaemia are often attributable to poor antenatal care. As the number of maternal deaths from all causes has declined, abortion has become relatively more important. The Abortion Act (1967) has brought about a substantial decrease in deaths from illegal operations and a small increase in deaths from legal abortion. The risk of coloured women dying of an illegal abortion is especially high.

In assessing obstetric achievement it is also essential to consider the results with the fetus or newborn child, of which the most useful indication is perinatal mortality. This index groups together stillbirths and deaths in the first week of life, both of which can be attributed broadly to influences operating before and during delivery. Figure 21 shows the trend of perinatal mortality in England and Wales since 1928 (when stillbirths were first registered) and compares it with the trend of mortality in the first month and the first year of life. While the decline of postneonatal deaths, mainly due to infections, has been much more impressive, the reduction of perinatal mortality has been considerable. This has not been attributable to advances in medical knowledge or obstetric services as specific as those which largely explain the decline of maternal mortality, but improvements in antenatal care and obstetric services have certainly made an important contribution.

Hospital or home confinement

There are wide differences of opinion about the desirability of conducting a substantial proportion of deliveries at home. In Sweden and the United States almost all doctors favour institutional delivery, and in New York, for example, 98 per cent of births are in hospital (the remaining 2 per cent are said to be in taxis).

Experience in countries such as England and the Netherlands shows that given good antenatal care, reasonable home conditions, well-trained midwives, and an efficient emergency service, domiciliary delivery is compatible with relatively low perinatal and maternal mortality rates. Yet there are grounds for believing that these rates might be even lower if all deliveries were in hospital. For when perinatal mortality is low further reduction depends on the skilful handling of problems which are technically complex and sometimes cannot be anticipated. The need cannot be met entirely by emergency measures in the home, nor by hasty transfer of a mother or new born child to hospital. It is mainly for this reason that most experienced obstetricians favour hospital confinement and also why we are moving rapidly towards a time when all deliveries will be conducted in hospital

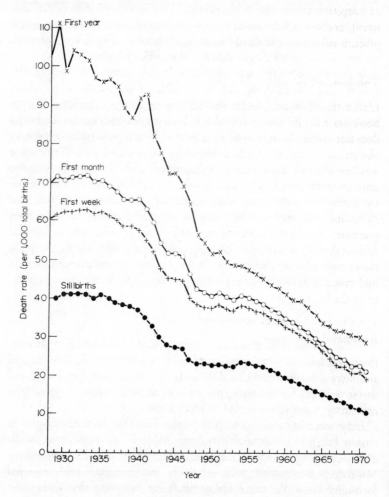

Figure 21. Death rate at birth and by end of first week, first month and first year.

or in short-stay general practitioner obstetric units. Although a maternity hospital is the safest place for the mother and her baby during and immediately after labour, a good home is undoubtedly the best place for a normal baby after the first few hours. The time when mother and child should be transferred from hospital to home is a matter for individual assessment, but in the majority of cases the transfer can be made within 12 to 48 hours. An increasing proportion of hospital obstetric beds are occupied for only 48 hours (short-stay units), and the small number of women who are cared for in general practitioner maternity units usually return home within 12 hours.

The general practitioner obstetrician

Under the National Health Service a woman may, without charge, book her own doctor to attend her during her confinement, and if he does not undertake midwifery she may choose a 'general-practitioner-obstetrician' from the local obstetric list. When the Act was framed it was intended that admission to the obstetric list should be granted only to practitioners who had shown a special interest in midwifery, by having held a resident, postgraduate appointment in obstetrics, or by having dealt with a certain number of midwifery cases in their own practices, but these requirements have not been strictly observed. Although the doctor engaged by a patient accepts full responsibility for the management of pregnancy, labour and puerperium, in practice the midwife is still the normal attendant at birth. However, in case of difficulty she has on call a medical attendant who should know the patient.

Antenatal supervision

In 1946 at least 80 per cent of women confined at home attended local authority antenatal clinics; today women rely on their general practitioner and the maternity hospital for antenatal supervision. The maternity medical service was intended to be an addition to facilities already available, not a substitute for them. Close supervision is required if the complications of pregnancy and labour are to be discovered early enough to avoid unnecessary morbidity and mortality. Most doctors recognize this but by no means all see their patients fortnightly until the thirtysixth week and then weekly until they are confined, as was the practice in local authority clinics. Moreover many services were more easily provided at a clinic than they are at a general practitioner's surgery, and clinics offered an excellent opportunity for instruction in preparation for childbirth, and for contact with the health visitor who would visit the home after the birth. The growing tendency for practitioners to practise in groups and from health centres makes it easier to provide a high standard of antenatal care.

Birth control and abortion

There is growing demand for a comprehensive and free family planning and birth control service as a normal part of the National Health Service. In 1969, the first full operational year of the Abortion Act, 54,157 women were legally aborted. In 1971 the number was 126,774 and the annual number is still rising. It is hoped that making contraceptive advice and prescriptions for contraceptives a regular part of the National Health Services will lessen the demand for abortion and discourage the use of abortion as a method of birth control.

FURTHER READING

Report on Confidential Enquiries into Maternal Deaths in England and Wales, 1967–69 (1972). D.H.S.S. Reports on Health and Social Subjects No. 1. H.M.S.O.

27 · SERVICES FOR CHILDREN

One quarter of the population of Britain is under the age of 16. In this chapter we are concerned with the special health needs of this important sector of the population and the health services that have evolved to meet those needs. From the point of view of needs, three age periods can be distinguished: the neonatal period; the post neonatal period (from the end of the first month to the end of the first year); and the rest of childhood through adolescence to school leaving.

We have already seen that most of the problems arising in the neonatal period are related to prenatal and intranatal influences (Chapter 2). The principal causes of death and disability are immaturity, malformation and birth injury. Prevention of these conditions, so far as they are preventable, lies largely in the province of the obstetric services, but the care of affected infants who survive into childhood calls for coordination of paediatric, nursing, social and educational services in hospital and community.

The post neonatal death rate remained very high until the beginning of the twentieth century, since when it has declined dramatically. Most of deaths were due to gastroenteritis, bronchitis and pneumonia, malnutrition, tuberculosis and the common infections of childhood (measles, whooping cough, diphtheria and scarlet fever). These causes of death are particularly susceptible to control by manipulation of adverse physical and social environments (bad feeding, lack of cleanliness, insanitary housing, overcrowding, maternal inefficiency, low standards of medical care) and the evolution of services to effect that manipulation has been largely responsible for the decline of the death rate. In recent years infant deaths have been the subject of confidential enquiries of the type previously undertaken only for maternal deaths. Retrospective enquiries are not easy to interpret, but the results indicate that there is still considerable scope for further reduction in the post neonatal death rate, mainly by raising the standards of care of low birthweight and sick new born babies and by paying more attention to the total situation of such infants in the post neonatal period—their vulnerability to infection and the adequacy of their parents and of the home environment. In particular, doctors, nurses and social workers need always to bear in mind the rapidity with which an ailing infant's condition can change for the worse.

From about the end of the first year children enter an extended period during which the risk of dying is extremely low. But although mortality is low, morbidity is comparatively high. Upper respiratory and bowel infections are common, and it is at this time that most of the common infections of childhood are contracted. By the age of 15, about four-fifths of children have had chickenpox, threequarters measles and whooping cough, and one-tenth scarlet fever. Rickets, bone and joint tuberculosis, rheumatic fever and diphtheria, all at one time common, are now rare, but accidents in the home and on the streets remain an important cause of morbidity and sometimes of permanent handicap. The period of childhood is also characterized by rapid growth and development and in the late years by the physical, psychological and social manifestations of adolesence. Health needs are determined by these characteristics. Children need a diet adequate to meet the demands of rapid growth, protection against infection and physical injury, a background conducive to normal social and emotional development, and surveillance to detect and where possible treat and correct congenital and acquired disabilities, with appropriate educational and social services in support.

With the reorganization of the National Health Service in 1974, school health services were transferred from local authorities to area health authorities. This for the first time placed all child health services within one administrative framework. However, because of the way in which services for children evolved and because the responsibility for educational and social services still rests with local authorities, it will be convenient to consider separately services for preschool children and services for school children.

PRESCHOOL CHILDREN

Hospital and general practitioner paediatrics

Hospital interest in diseases of children is even more recent than in obstetrics. The provision of special hospitals for such children began as a voluntary movement in the middle of the nineteenth century (Great Ormond Street Hospital was founded in 1852) and remained largely a voluntary matter until the National Health Service. Many workhouse inmates were young children, but until well into the twentieth century special accommodation for children in public hospitals was limited to fever hospitals. Paediatrics is now a well developed specialty and most of the children in district general hospitals are gathered together in children's departments with appropriate facilities (open visiting, sleeping accommodation for mothers, day rooms and play areas). Like other well developed specialties it is already fragmenting into sub-specialties—perinatal paediatrics, developmental paediatrics, paediatric cardiology, gastroenterology, neurology, oncology, haematology.

During the nineteenth and early part of the twentieth centuries, deficiencies in medical education and lack of financial incentive kept the standard of general practitioner paediatrics at a low level. Academic instruction in paediatrics was first given by obstetricians, and it was not until the second half of the nineteenth century that medical schools began to show any real interest in the subject. The first chair was established in 1906 (King's College, London), and it was said in London that the only thing most doctors knew about the care of children was Dr. Still's telephone number. It was not until the Second World War that universities began to put the subject on an equal footing with medicine, surgery and midwifery in the final examination.

The National Health Insurance Act of 1911 provided the first public domiciliary medical service (outside the Poor Law), but it made no arrangements for the children of insured workers. Some doctors accepted children in sick clubs, and for a few pence per week contracted to provide medicine and advice when needed. Nevertheless the medical care of preschool children remained most unsatisfactory until the National Health Service made available without charge a general practitioner service for every child.

Local authority services

When local authorities entered the field of personal health services at the beginning of the century in response to public concern about the inadequacy of provisions for the care of children, the voluntary infant welfare movement comprised three main activities:

1. Home visiting for the purpose of advising recently confined mothers on the feeding, clothing and general care of their children. This was the British contribution to the infant welfare movement and the origin of the Health Visiting Service. It began in Manchester in 1862, first on a voluntary basis and later as a salaried service.

2. Consultation clinics, introduced in France ('consultations de nourrisons'), for medical supervision of children which were in effect the first child welfare centres.

3. Distribution through milk depots ('goutes de lait') of cheap, safe milk to mothers not able to breast feed their babies, also first developed in France.

These features were gradually adopted and developed by local authorities. From them evolved the child welfare service which Local Health Authorities provided under the National Health Service, the responsibility for which now rests with Area Health Authorities.

(a) *Health visiting*

In the past there was great variation in the qualifications and experience of health visitors, who at different times and in different places have been voluntary 'lady visitors', working class women with families of their own who had undergone a short course of instruction, sanitary inspectors, midwives, nurses and even doctors. Today only state registered nurses with training in midwifery are accepted for the twelve months full time training which leads to the Certificate in Health Visiting.

The health visitor calls on the mother within a few days of her return home from hospital, or, in the case of early discharge or home delivery, as soon as possible after the midwife has left. She has no legal right of entry but is rarely refused admission. After the first visit she encourages the mother to attend an infant welfare centre, but she visits the home again from time to time as she thinks necessary. Although she is a trained nurse, she does not undertake sick-nursing duties, except occasionally in rural areas. Her province is to advise and educate the mother with regard to such matters as maintenance of breast feeding, preparation of artificial feeds, weaning and protection of the child against infection and accident. In short she is concerned with the control of the domestic environment to reduce the risks of death and disability. Although health visitors still have an important role in the care of expectant and nursing mothers and of children under 5 years of age, their field of interest has been extended greatly by the National Health Service Act and by general practitioner attachment schemes. They now give advice about health problems affecting other members of the family, particularly the elderly, the sick and the handicapped.

(b) *Child welfare centres*

The original purpose of child welfare centres was to follow up the progress of preschool children under medical and health visitor supervision. From the beginning many centres provided food for mothers and children at reduced rates (free in necessitous cases). Later cod liver oil was also dispensed. Since the closing of the Ministry of Food (after the Second World War) local health authorities have accepted responsibility for the distribution of National Dried Milk and vitamin supplements. Proprietary foods are still often available at wholesale prices on the recommendation of the doctor, and the distribution of food is considered by some to provide an important incentive for attendance.

The centres are now the focal point for medical consultation and for advice and education about all matters related to the health of young children. They provide facilities for screening for defects of vision and hearing, assessment of child development and early diagnosis and assessment of physical and mental handicaps.

Most of the doctors who work in the centres are women. They may be full time medical officers on the staff of the Area Health Authority or may attend on a sessional basis (in which case they may be also in general practice or in hospital paediatric practice) and they usually have postgraduate experience in developmental paediatrics, child psychiatry and clinical paediatrics. When a child first attends a centre, usually between two and six weeks of age, it is examined by the doctor. Subsequent examinations, at six months and then approximately at each birthday up to the age of four, are tending to become a responsibility shared between doctor and health visitor. The health visitor assumes the role of observer in the early detection of handicaps and is often made responsible for screening tests. In this respect the attachment of health visitors to group general practices, especially in health centres, has great advantages for communications and access to records.

Appraisal of services for preschool children

The development of child welfare centres with their three services—health education, medical examination and food distribution—coincided with a rapid decline in child mortality, but in the same period there were other changes likely to improve the health of children, for example, a decrease in mean family size, improvement in the standard of living, and, more recently, the introduction of effective therapy. We must therefore rely on a commonsense appraisal of each type of service.

There can be little doubt that the instruction of an uninformed mother by an experienced health visitor or doctor is valuable. Breast feeding, bowel-training, preparation of artificial foods, and weaning are not matters in which it is possible to rely either on a mothers' instinctive good sense, or on the advice given by friends or relatives. A few women in favourable circumstances have received suitable instruction from other sources, mainly from private doctors, but most women have obtained it from welfare centres or not at all. However, much of the traditional advisory work of doctors in welfare centres can now be done equally well by the health visitor. Indeed the conditions for which medical advice is given are those with which the health visitor has been trained to deal, and does deal when no doctor is available.

The initial medical examination is a different matter. This demands more knowledge of developmental paediatrics and a wider knowledge of congenital defects and clinical medicine than the health visitor can command. Subsequent surveillance of young children's developmental and health progress can probably be left to health visitors provided they have facilities for early referral to doctors with a special interest in and knowledge of child health. Such doctors in their turn need the backing of comprehensive multidisciplinary assessment centres for handicapped children of the type that teaching hospitals are now beginning to establish.

The importance of the contribution that the distribution of dried milk and vitamin supplements from welfare centres has made to the health of young children is not in doubt. However, it is to be hoped that in the future the reputation of welfare centres will rest on the high quality of their work, and it is difficult to see how the sale of infant foods does anything to enhance that reputation and this should be organized as a separate activity.

The personal health services of local authorities were introduced because of concern about the health of children at a time when infectious disease was predominant. When one child in ten was dying from an infection in the first year of life, the most urgent requirement was to protect those who were normal at birth from the deleterious effects of the postnatal environment. Children died mainly because they were underfed and because they were infected at a vulnerable age in overcrowded and insanitary homes. It was in such circumstances that the domiciliary services for children developed, with the health visitor as the key worker. Her job was not to nurse the sick child, but to attempt to prevent sickness by advice and assistance to the mother.

In decaying areas of cities there are still underprivileged children and families who have to be made aware of and persuaded to use available services. However, with higher standards of living, a better educated population and comprehensive medical services, the health of the normal child has become more secure and the problems of children who are physically or mentally handicapped have become relatively more important.

The health visitor is well placed for the early ascertainment of handicaps. She is the only health worker who sees all children soon after birth and at intervals during early life. Her experience in dealing with the health problems of mothers and young children is unrivalled. Now that the earlier objectives of her work have been largely achieved, the policy of attaching health visitors to groups of general practitioners is a natural development, with a shift in emphasis from an advisory role to one focussed on ascertaining and helping the sick and handicapped of all ages.

SCHOOL CHILDREN

Local authority services

Compulsory education was introduced in 1870, but widespread malnutrition interfered with the proper use of this facility and in 1906 an education act permitted the new local education authorities to provide milk and meals to elementary school children who were unable by reason of lack of food to take full advantage of the education provided for them. At about the same time the Interdepartmental Committee on Physical Deterioration recommended that 'a systematized inspection of school children should be imposed as a public duty on every school authority' and this led to another education act in 1907 which laid the foundations for a school health service. Regular medical inspections soon revealed a substantial amount of untreated illness and disability among the children, and local education authorities began to provide treatment in clinics, first for minor ailments such as skin conditions and later for ophthalmological, orthopaedic and other conditions. Medical inspections also helped to identify children with serious physical and mental handicaps who needed special educational treatment.

(a) *Milk and meals*

The provision of milk and meals by local education authorities was for a long time an inadequate and unattractive service subject to a means test. The upheaval of the war of 1939-45 changed its character —many mothers were out at work and the need to maintain the health of children led to a great expansion of the service and freed it of its association with poverty. Free milk is now provided for children at nursery schools, for handicapped pupils and, where there are medical reasons, for junior school pupils. The uptake of school meals, for which there is a small charge, is high and there is a movement towards providing cafeteria, free-choice meals for older pupils. It is a sign of our affluent times that medical interest in the nutrition of school children has moved from the problems of under nutrition to those of obesity and dental caries.

(b) *Medical inspections*

School inspections were introduced to identify previously unrecognized defects in children, to supervise their treatment and to ensure that serious defects impeded educational progress as little as possible. They provided, in fact, a screening programme for school children long before screening became fashionable. With the developments in the preschool services, a national health service and a growing interest in developmental paediatrics most of the defects likely to interfere with education are now discovered and well-documented before school entry, but the surveillance of preschool children is still not sufficiently comprehensive for the school entry medical examination to be dispensed with. At that examination a child's medical history, physical growth, vision, hearing, speech, motor function and intellectual, social and emotional development are reassessed in the learning situation. Subsequent examinations are much more selective—special examinations at the request of parents, teacher, school nurse or health visitor. The role of the school nurse was at one time limited to receptionist and cleanliness inspector at the routine medical examinations. It is now being extended to include tests of visual and auditory acuity and of physical and neuromotor development.

(c) *School clinics*

Under the Education Act of 1944 local education authorities were required to provide, free of cost to parents, all forms of treatment (except domiciliary treatment) for pupils attending maintained schools. This treatment was provided in minor ailment clinics and specialist clinics. The clinics offered treatment for a wide range of conditions (ophthalmic, orthopaedic, otolaryngological) and many special services (speech therapy, child guidance, remedial exercises, orthoptic services). Formerly the clinics were staffed and maintained by local education authorities but under the National Health Service they became the responsibility first of Regional Hospital Boards and now of Area Health Authorities. There is a growing tendency to transfer the specialist services from the clinics to hospital out-patients departments.

(d) *Handicapped children*

Seriously handicapped children often have special educational needs and sometimes those needs can be met satisfactorily only in special schools. It is the statutory duty of local education authorities to 'ascertain' such children and to provide special educational facilities for them in ordinary or special schools (Chapters 28 and 29).

Appraisal of services

Over the past century mortality rates have declined more for children than for any other age group. They have fallen to the extent that in

1971 the death rate for children aged 5-14 was less than one-twentieth of the rate in 1841-50. Almost all of this improvement is due to the decline of mortality from infectious disease attributable mainly to a rising standard of living, control of unhygienic living conditions and, latterly, immunization programmes.

The general health of children has also improved a great deal, although this is not so well documented (despite the routine recording for more than sixty years of defects found at routine school medical inspections). There has certainly been a remarkable increase in the height and weight of children and decrease in the mean age at onset of menstruation in girls. On the average children aged twelve years are 4 inches taller and 10 pounds heavier than children of the same age sixty years ago and girls begin to menstruate three years earlier than they did at the beginning of the century. Skin, eye and ear infections are much less common and rickets and bone and joint tuberculosis have become extremely rare conditions. It is impossible to assess reliably the contribution of the school health services to this improvement in health, but it is safe to say that they have been less important than the rising standard of living, improvement in environmental services and introduction of immunization procedures. Even the provision of milk and meals at school can have had no very great effect before the Second World War, for the milk in schools scheme was not introduced until 1934 and in 1938 only 4 per cent of children were taking school meals. Since then, however, school meals, the treatment of major and minor ailments and disabilities and the medical surveillance of sub-groups of handicapped children in relation to their educational progress must have made an increasingly important contribution.

Routine school inspections, school dinners and school medical officers of the old type are now an anachronism and are fast disappearing. But there is no question about the continuing need for the following:

1. Surveillance of the physical growth and the educational, social and emotional development of all children attending school;

2. Identification of children with physical or mental defects which may affect their ability to learn in the ordinary school situation;

3. Continued medical surveillance of children with physical and mental disorders which may have important implications for their educational and psychological development;

4. Advice for teachers to help them to interpret the educational significance of what doctors may know about particular children;

5. A multidisciplinary consultation service for children with educational problems that may have underlying physical, social or psychological causes and for adolescents with difficulties in relation to psychosexual adjustment, drug taking and other health matters;

6. Maintenance of immunization programmes for school children;

7. An advisory service on health education programmes in schools.

Services to meet those needs have in the past developed under the auspices of local authorities. It remains to be seen how they will be coordinated and administered now that they have been made the responsibility of Area Health Authorities. For the first time in our social history one authority is responsible for all preschool and school child health services. This provides a unique opportunity to develop a fully integrated child health service.

FURTHER READING

Confidential Enquiry into Postneonatal Deaths 1964–66 (1970). D.H.S.S. Reports on Public Health and Medical Subjects No. 125. H.M.S.O.

COURT D. and JACKSON A. (eds.) (1972) *Paediatrics in the Seventies.* Nuffield Provincial Hospitals Trust. Oxford University Press.

28 · SERVICES FOR THE PHYSICALLY HANDICAPPED

The significance of physical handicaps is determined much more by their social consequences and by personal and public attitudes to them than by their medical description. Although this implies that the needs of handicapped persons are essentially social in character, it does not mean that they are of no concern to doctors. Without the cooperation of the medical profession, the services provided to help handicapped people cannot function properly: the health services provide treatment and medical rehabilitation; and medical opinion is required about prognosis and any limitations that should be imposed on physical activity.

The significance of handicaps in children depends upon the extent to which they interfere with physical, emotional, social and, above all, educational development. In adults important considerations are the restrictions the handicaps impose on ability to lead an independent social life—to work, to marry and to enjoy a normal family life.

PHYSICALLY HANDICAPPED CHILDREN

Broadly speaking there are two ways in which a physical handicap may disturb family life: it may require separation of the affected child from parents, brothers and sisters because of the need for hospital treatment or for educational facilities that can be provided only in a residential school; and it may have an adverse effect upon the mental or physical health of other members of the family.

There are also two ways in which a handicap may influence the course of education. On the one hand it may be of such a nature that the child cannot be educated by normal methods, as, for example, in the case of blind and deaf children and children with gross spastic defects. Here the difficulties are mainly educational. On the other hand a physical handicap, although in no way affecting educability, may make it difficult or impossible for a child to attend an ordinary school. For example a child may be in hospital undergoing protracted surgical treatment or may be unable to meet the physical demands of school life because of congenital heart disease. Such difficulties are essentially medical.

Until the present century, responsibility for the welfare and education of physically disabled children rested almost entirely with parents. Most of the crippling disabilities of childhood (rickets, bone and joint tuberculosis, and blindness and deafness due to infection in infancy) were directly related to a low standard of living, and a handicapped child, if too disabled to work on the land or in a factory, remained neglected at home or, if abandoned by its family, was admitted to the general mixed workhouse.

In the eighteenth century voluntary effort had begun to prepare the way for a more humane public approach, but the services provided were inevitably local and limited in scope. For the most part they were concerned with the welfare and training of the two groups of children whose disabilities have always aroused sympathy: the blind (first school established in Liverpool, 1792); and the deaf and dumb (first school, Edinburgh 1760). The needs of children with less appealing disabilities were largely ignored.

With the introduction of compulsory education (1870) and the subsequent development of school health services, the extent of the need for special educational facilities to help severely disabled children to compensate for their handicaps was slowly uncovered. Appropriate services developed slowly and it is only since the Education Act, 1944, that an attempt has been made to ensure that all severely handicapped children receive an education suited to their 'age, ability and aptitude'. Under the act local education authorities are statutorily responsible for 'ascertaining' all the children in their areas who are likely to need specialized educational facilities and for providing those facilities.

If some concession is made to their special needs (for example a seat at the front of the class for a child with defective sight or hearing), children with moderate handicaps can often attend an ordinary school. This is undoubtedly the best place for them. Unfortunately most severely handicapped children lose a great deal of time from school for medical reasons, and their educational progress tends to be slower than that of other children of their own age. To help them in their unequal struggle they need a great deal of individual attention and sometimes this can be provided only in a special class, in a special school (which may be of day or residential type), or in hospital.

Regulations made under the Education Act, 1944, define ten categories of children needing special educational treatment: the blind, the partially sighted, the deaf, the partially hearing, the educationally subnormal, the epileptic, the maladjusted, the physically handicapped, children with speech defect, and the delicate. Estimates of the incidence of these disabilities in the population of school children depend on definition, completeness of ascertainment and availability of the appropriate special education facilities. Table 25 provides a working estimate of the size of the contemporary problem in terms of the children requiring and receiving special educational treatment in 1971. For convenience maladjusted children are mentioned in this chapter, but the needs of mentally subnormal children are discussed in Chapter 29.

Blind and partially sighted children

For educational purposes blind children are defined as those with no sight or whose sight is, or is likely to become, so defective that they require education by methods not involving the use of sight. Partially sighted children are those who by reason of defective vision cannot follow the ordinary curriculum without detriment to their sight or to their educational development, but can be educated by special methods involving sight. At the present time about 3,650 children of school age (5 per 10,000) have such poor vision that they are unable to read ordinary school books; 2,400 of them can be taught by visual methods with the help of magnifying glasses and specially printed books, but the education of the rest depends upon non-visual methods. It is the practice to meet the needs of the partially sighted so far as possible in ordinary schools, reserving special residential schools for the blind. When the defect is stable (congenital cataract, dislocated lens, corneal scarring after injury or infection) educational classification can be based on tests of visual acuity after full correction. When the defect is progressive the educational decision is more difficult, and rests upon a medical estimate of whether or not the sight is likely to deteriorate beyond the point at which education by visual methods

Table 25. Children receiving and requiring special education treatment: England and Wales 1971

Number of children:	Blind	Partially sighted	Deaf	Partially Hearing	Physically Handi- capped	Delicate	Maladjusted	Educa- tionally Subnormal	Epileptic	Speech Defects	Total
Receiving special educational treatment	1,141	2,204	3,817	4,450	11,316	7,797	12,669	58,012	806	286	102,498
Requiring special treatment but not yet placed	91	218	121	204	741	679	1,865	10,114	53	93	14,179
Total	1,232	2,422	3,938	4,654	12,057	8,476	14,534	68,126	859	379	116,677*
Rate per 10,000 children of school-age	1·6	3·1	5·1	6·0	15·6	10·9	18·7	87·8	1·1	0·4	150·3

* Excludes 3,537 pupils on the registers of hospital special schools.

will become impossible. For example the commonest cause of progressive visual deterioration in childhood is now myopia and in the great majority of cases this is progressive only until growth is complete; in a small proportion of cases with choroidal and retinal degeneration the visual defect progresses to blindness and if these children are to come to terms with their tragic disability the sooner they are taught to read by touch the better.

Deaf and partially hearing children

Deaf children are defined as those whose hearing is so defective that they require education by methods used for pupils with little or no naturally acquired speech or language. Partially hearing children are those whose hearing is so defective that they require for their education special arrangements or facilities, but not all the educational methods used for deaf pupils.

The introduction of audiometry into routine preschool and school examinations has uncovered a great deal of previously unsuspected deafness—about one in twentyfive children tested has an appreciable auditory impairment in both ears. With a little extra attention in the classroom, tuition in lip reading, the provision of suitable hearing aids and the treatment of chronic ear infection, the needs of the great majority of these children can be met in ordinary schools. However, nine in every ten thousand school children have an auditory defect serious enough to need special educational facilities. Auditory handicap is therefore twice as common as visual handicap although it excites considerably less public sympathy. Today most children classified as deaf are born with their handicap. It must be remembered, however, that congenital deafness is not necessarily or indeed usually genetic in origin; in some cases it is attributable to environmental influences such as maternal rubella, birth injury, anoxia and rhesus incompatibility.

The education of deaf children presents formidable problems, and their long and difficult training must begin very early in life if they are to be taught to speak intelligibly. Early ascertainment is therefore of the utmost importance.

Epileptic children

Epilepsy is a common condition—about four per thousand children of school age are known to be under treatment for it. Fortunately, the great majority of these children are able to attend and make satisfactory progress in ordinary schools. In 1971 only 859 epileptic children (one in ten thousand of the school population) were receiving education in special schools, two thirds of them in residential schools. Very frequent and severe fits, marked behavioural difficulties and lack of educational progress determine the need for special schooling.

Maladjusted children

Maladjusted children are pupils who show evidence of emotional instability or psychological disturbance, and who require special educational treatment in order to effect their personal, social or educational readjustment. The causes of maladjustment are complex and imperfectly understood. The tense emotional atmosphere in homes with marital difficulties, the antipathy that sometimes develops between parent and child and the overcrowding and lack of playing space in the poorer parts of industrial towns are a few of the many influences thought to lie behind the antisocial behaviour (destructiveness, lying, stealing, etc.) of some children. Children with physical handicaps, with chronic or recurrent illness or with a poor intellectual endowment may also present behaviour problems which can become serious if handled impatiently or with lack of understanding by parents, teachers and doctors.

A child guidance service is now provided in most areas by a team consisting of a psychiatrist, an educational psychologist and a psychiatric social worker. But the service is time consuming and costly, the demands upon it are heavy and waiting lists tend to be long. There are also special residential schools to which the most seriously disturbed children can be sent for a period of observation and treatment, although bringing together children of very different types and often with conflicting needs has obvious dangers.

Physically handicapped children

These are pupils who are not suffering from a defect of sight or hearing but who by reason of disease or crippling defect cannot, without detriment to their health or educational development, be satisfactorily educated under the normal regime of ordinary schools.

In 1971 about 12,000 pupils were classified as physically handicapped and were being educated in special classes, day schools and boarding schools. The types of children included under this broad heading are so diverse and their needs so varied that it is difficult to make any worthwhile generalization about them.

In recent years cerebral palsy has been the commonest cause of severe physical handicap, but since about 1970 the number of children with spina bifida in many special schools now equals or exceeds the number with cerebral palsy. Neonatal surgery has improved the chances of survival of infants with meningomyelocele but the quality of survival is often a matter for regret, and for parents a cause of great distress. Assessment of the medical, social and educational needs of the survivors presents a difficult interdisciplinary problem as it can involve neurosurgeon, urologist, orthopaedic surgeon, paediatrician, general practitioner, school health physician, medical social worker, health visitor, educational psychologist and teacher.

In the past children most seriously affected with cerebral palsy were regarded as ineducable, and from poorer homes they often found their way into institutions for the mentally defective. Since 1940 many special schools, training centres and clinics have been opened for these unfortunate children, with encouraging results. Other crippling handicaps also present special problems (muscular dystrophy, congenital heart disease and limb deformities, rheumatic heart disease), but surgical techniques and the design of surgical appliances have advanced so rapidly in recent years that many of even the more severely handicapped children eventually become self supporting.

Children with speech defects

Speech defects are very common in childhood—it has been stated that two per cent of school children would benefit from treatment by a speech therapist. However, the number of children with such defects who require special schooling is extremely small; the great majority are able to continue with their ordinary schooling while their disability is being assessed and treated. There is at present such a serious shortage of speech therapists that few local education authorities are able to meet the demand for their services.

Delicate children

These are children who do not fall into any of the previous categories but who by reason of impaired physical condition need a change of environment or cannot, without risk to their health and educational progress, be educated in ordinary schools. They include children in poor health from many causes including bad home conditions (lack of sleep and faulty feeding), and children debilitated from asthma and other illnesses or operations. What is usually needed is a period of convalescence under medical supervision, with good food, fresh air and plenty of rest, and a programme of teaching which enables them to progress for a while at a slower educational pace. To meet those needs an extensive system of open air schools has been developed over the past fifty years. The demand for such accommodation is declining but is still substantial. About three-quarters of the accommodation is provided in day schools to which the children are taken in special buses. On the average children are kept on the register of a day school for from eighteen months to two years. The rest of the accommodation is provided in residential schools in which the children rarely stay for more than six months.

Appraisal of services for physically handicapped children

Effective planning must take into account past trends as well as current needs if future requirements are to be met, and like the pattern of mortality, the pattern of disability in childhood has undergone a remarkable change during the sixty years since the school health services began. As we have seen, this change has been characterized by a decline in the incidence of disability due to adverse postnatal environmental influences (in particular malnutrition and infection) with the result that disability due to natal and prenatal (including genetic) influences has become increasingly prominent. This is particularly obvious in the case of blindness and physical disability.

At the beginning of the nineteenth century two thirds of those applying for relief at the Liverpool School for the Indigent Blind were thought to have lost their sight because of smallpox. By the end of the century smallpox had virtually disappeared, and the Ophthalmological Society of the United Kingdom estimated that a third or more of the inmates of blind schools had lost their sight because of ophthalmia neonatorum. Nowadays the contribution of infection to the pool of blindness in school children is negligible, and congenital defects, myopia, diseases of the central nervous system and tumours together account for more than 80 per cent of all cases. Associated with this change in the pattern of causes of blindness has been a steady decline in the number of children requiring special educational facilities. Between 1923 and 1971 the number of school children registered as blind in England fell from 2,723 to 1,252. (After 1955 there was a sharp but temporary increase as a cohort of children with retrolental fibroplasia moved through the blind schools. This condition was caused by intensive administration of oxygen to premature infants from about 1947 to 1958.)

The causes and the incidence of physically crippling disease in childhood have changed in much the same way. At the beginning of the present century rickets, bone and joint tuberculosis, rheumatic heart disease and osteomyelitis were the principal causes of disablement. Rickets as a cause of deformity has disappeared, osteomyelitis and bone and joint tuberculosis are no longer of any importance, and rheumatic heart disease is far less common. In the immediate post war period there was a temporary increase in the amount of disablement due to poliomyelitis. The number of cases notified between 1945 and 1956 was between 2,000 and 8,000 a year. But with the introduction of effective vaccines, the numbers have declined sharply and since 1969 the annual number of notifications has been less than ten. With the decline of infections, there has been a substantial reduction in the overall incidence of severe disablement, and cerebral palsy, spina bifida, congenital heart disease and asthma are now major causes of crippling in childhood.

Paradoxically, as special services for handicapped children have developed the need for them has declined. With the rising standard of living and even more effective control of the common infections of childhood and their complications, it seems fairly certain that the incidence of serious disablement in childhood will decline still further. At the same time with smaller classes and more modern buildings and equipment many more handicapped children can be given the benefit of an education in an ordinary school. Although more refined, elaborate and expensive educational services are likely to be introduced to deal with the hard core of serious disablement which will remain, it seems likely that the demand for and cost of special schools will be further reduced before the end of the century.

The separation of handicapped children into mutually exclusive categories has had its uses but it is no longer very acceptable. So many children, whatever their main physical disability, have multiple handicaps. The assessment and fostering of each child's physical and intellectual assets is more important than the definition of a leading disability. Many more multidisciplinary assessment centres are needed, but there is a danger that the fragmentation of hospital paediatrics into an increasing number of sub-specialties may tend to work against this trend.

PHYSICALLY HANDICAPPED ADULTS

Adults with a handicap which intereferes with their ability to work may be grouped as follows:

(a) Those handicapped since childhood (e.g. the congenitally blind). For this group special educational facilities and expert guidance during the transition from school to work are of outstanding importance.

(b) Those with a temporary disability (e.g. respiratory tuberculosis). Here the need is for efficient and well coordinated medical rehabilitation services to reduce the period of incapacity and to enable the worker to return, if possible, to his previous occupation.

(c) Those who acquire a permanent handicap (e.g. the loss of a limb) but are still capable of employment in open industry. In this group industrial rehabilitation is the paramount need. A change of occupation is often necessary, so retraining and help in finding suitable employment may be called for.

(d) Those with a permanent disability so incapacitating that although capable of some work they may never be fit for ordinary employment (for example gross rheumatoid arthritis). The need of this group is for work under sheltered and supervised conditions.

(e) Those with a permanent, and often progressive handicap (e.g. advanced disseminated sclerosis) which for practical purposes makes them unsuitable for any employment. In this group the first need is for adequate medical and nursing care, preferably at home, but if this is not possible, in an institution. Any occupation will be mainly diversional.

Evolution of services

Except under the Poor Law, there were no public services for handicapped adults before the end of the nineteenth century. In 1897 the Workman's Compensation Act recognized some financial obligation to persons injured at work, and in 1911 the National Health Insurance

Act offered general practititioner care for sick and disabled workers in the lower wage ranges. But it is only recently that an attempt has been made to provide comprehensive services to help seriously disabled persons to find and keep suitable employment.

The two World Wars played a significant part in arousing public interest and compelling national action. In 1914-18 an attempt was made to reduce the serious loss of manpower due to badly treated gunshot wounds (and in particular those associated with fractures) by setting up rehabilitation centres in military hospitals. Immediately after the war public sympathy for permanently disabled ex-service men (notably for the blind) led to the establishment of Government Instructional Factories to retrain them and to the introduction of the King's National Roll scheme to encourage firms to employ them. The idea of medical rehabilitation for the injured took root and became an accepted, if inadequate, part of hospital practice. But the feeling of urgency about the need to find employment for the disabled was soon dissipated, and apart from some improvement in services for the blind, no further progress was made until the Second World War. Then the acute shortage of manpower, both in the armed forces and in industry, led to a considerable expansion of medical rehabilitation services in hospitals and to the introduction of a national service for non-medical rehabilitation and resettlement under the Disabled Persons (Employment) Acts of 1944 and 1958.

Contemporary services

Medical responsibility for the care of a patient incapacitated by illness or injury extends far beyond the immediate problem of diagnosis and treatment and can be said to end only when that patient is once more able to lead a reasonably independent social life. This demands from the doctor an appreciation of the effects of pathology upon function, and in particular upon ability to work and to perform the personal activities of daily life (washing, dressing, eating, getting up and downstairs, etc.). It requires from the hospitals a medical rehabilitation service that will minimize disability.

For the patient rehabilitation should be a continuous process. But present day services for the handicapped have such complex ramifications that it will help to clarify their pattern if they are described under four headings: medical rehabilitation; industrial rehabilitation; welfare services; and services for young persons.

Medical rehabilitation

At most large hospitals a senior member of the medical staff is now responsible for rehabilitation services, which include physiotherapy, remedial gymnastics and occupational therapy. Therapy may be directed towards the strengthening of a particular function, or it may have the more general purpose of restoring physical and mental confidence after illness or injury. As we have indicated, such services were in the first place designed to meet the needs of the war injured; they are now used to great advantage in a wide range of medical and surgical conditions, including diseases and injuries of the central nervous system (poliomyelitis, paraplegia, hemiplegia), chest conditions (asthma, bronchitis) and after thoracic and abdominal operations.

The aim of medical rehabilitation is to shorten the period between serious accident or illness and return to independent life in the community. For most men this means return to work; but for many women it means return to domestic responsibilities, and a number of hospitals now provide special rehabilitation services for disabled housewives.

For hospital rehabilitation services to be fully effective, regular conferences between medical staff, social workers and disablement resettlement officers (see over) are essential. Inadequately supervised and badly coordinated services can delay return to work by unnecessarily prolonging the need for attendance at hospital.

Industrial rehabilitation

Public responsibility for helping a disabled person to overcome the difficulty experienced in 'obtaining or keeping employment of a kind which apart from his injury, disease or deformity would be suited to his age, experience and qualifications' is now accepted by the Department of Employment under the Disabled Persons (Employment) Acts, 1944 and 1958. The services fall under five headings:

(a) Disabled persons' register

Application for registration, which is voluntary, is made at the local employment exchange. When the disability is obvious (e.g. loss of a limb) no medical certificate is required; in other cases confirmation from hospital or general practitioner may be asked for. There is an obligation on employers with twenty or more employees to employ 3 per cent of registered disabled, and certain occupations (lift and car park attendant) are 'designated' (reserved) for the disabled. The principal causes of disablement among those registered in 1972 are shown in table 26.

Table 26. Disabilities among registered disabled persons, April 1972

Nature of disability	Number	Percentage
Surgical Conditions		
Amputations	37,784	6·2
Injuries, etc. of lower limbs	76,590	12·5
Injuries, etc. of upper limbs	50,475	8·3
Injuries, etc. of head, neck and trunk	84,635	13·9
Medical Conditions		
Cardiovascular disease	64,183	10·5
Chronic bronchitis	49,831	8·2
Pulmonary tuberculosis	17,819	2·9
Pneumoconiosis	6,267	1·1
Arthritis and rheumatism	26,484	4·3
Digestive disease	18,692	3·1
Epilepsy	22,016	3·6
Other	31,875	5·2
Psychiatric Conditions	37,570	6·1
Eye and Ear Defects and Other Conditions	85,886	14·1
Total	610,107	100%

(b) Disablement resettlement officer

From each employment exchange the Department of Employment provides a specialist placing service operated through a disablement resettlement officer (D.R.O.) who advises disabled persons about registration and helps them to find suitable employment or, if necessary, arranges for them to attend courses of rehabilitation or vocational training. The D.R.O. has detailed knowledge of local working conditions and occupational opportunities and of the physical and mental demands that particular jobs make. He also keeps in close touch with employers and hospitals in his area.

(c) Industrial rehabilitation units

There are now twentyfive industrial rehabilitation units in the country. One unit is fully residential and two others have some residential accommodation for men. At non-residential units, persons who are unable to travel daily from home are found accommodation in lodgings

Table 27. Admissions to industrial rehabilitation units during 1971

Nature of disability	Number	Percentage
Surgical Conditions		
Amputations	279	1·9
Injuries, etc. of lower limbs	1,080	7·7
Injuries, etc. of upper limbs	651	4·6
Injuries, etc. of head, neck and trunk	2,042	14·6
Medical Conditions		
Cardiovascular disease	1,319	9·4
Respiratory disease	910	6·5
Pulmonary tuberculosis	166	1·2
Arthritis and rheumatism	367	2·6
Digestive disease	355	2·5
Epilepsy	627	4·5
Others	898	6·4
Mental Disorders	3,038	21·6
Eye and Ear Defects and other Conditions	1,302	9·2
No obvious disability	838	5·9
Left before examined	146	1·4
Total	14,018	100%

or hostels. Industrial rehabilitation units do not offer training for specific occupations: their purpose is to provide individual rehabilitation under conditions approximating to those in industry (hours of work, etc.) for disabled persons who, although no longer requiring medical treatment, are not yet fit to stand the strain of normal full-time employment. During 1971 over 14,000 men and women were admitted to the units (table 27). About 11,600 completed the courses, and 50 per cent of them were in work or had been accepted for training within three months of completion. Orthopaedic conditions (including those due to injury) account for about a quarter of all admissions, and psychoneurosis, psychosis and mental subnormality together account for another fifth.

Each unit is directed by a Rehabilitation Officer, and the staff consists of a Vocational Officer (an occupational psychologist responsible for assessing occupational aptitudes), a Social Worker to help the disabled with personal problems, a Chief Occupational Supervisor in charge of the workshops and a Disablement Resettlement Officer who is responsible for finding suitable employment at the end of the course. Medical advice and supervision are provided by the Employment Medical Advisory Service (Chapter 18).

(d) Government training centres

Intensive training courses of from six to twelve months are provided by the Department of Employment in more than fifty skilled and semi-skilled occupations at thirty government training centres. Although now mainly concerned with retraining the able-bodied these courses are also available for disabled persons, and some of the centres are situated alongside or are in the same building as industrial rehabilitation units. The training is costly, so applicants are not accepted unless there is reasonable prospect that at the end of their course they will be fit to enter the trade for which they have been trained and to stand up to normal working conditions.

(e) Sheltered employment

Some disabled persons are so severely handicapped that they are unlikely ever to obtain employment in open industry. To meet their needs a non-profit distributing (and also, it must be admitted, non-profit making) company, Remploy, was set up by the Ministry of Labour in 1945 under the Disabled Persons (Employment) Act. The first Remploy factory was opened at Bridgend, Glamorgan. Today about 7,600 severely disabled men and women are employed in 87 Remploy factories. Their disabilities are due to such conditions as advanced rheumatoid arthritis, disseminated sclerosis and chronic bronchitis. Remploy products are very varied, and include furniture, books (printing and binding), knitwear and orthopaedic equipment.

In addition to the Department of Employment's Remploy factories, there are also sheltered workshops run by the major local authorities, and by voluntary organizations such as the National Institute for the Blind.

Welfare services

With the help of rehabilitation and resettlement services many disabled adults are now able to find work which gives them economic independence. However, there are some so severely handicapped that they can never become economically self supporting, and a few need almost continuous care and attention. Responsibility for their welfare rests largely with the major local authorities under Part II of the National Assistance Act, 1948 (Part I is concerned with financial assistance for those whose needs are not met by National Insurance or other sources). Their responsibilities begin with ascertainment 'of persons who are blind, deaf or dumb, and other persons who are substantially and permanently handicapped by illness, injury or congenital deformity' with the purpose of assessing their social and welfare needs and making arrangements to meet those needs. The services include home visiting, clubs, outings, holiday homes, transport to and from home, sheltered workshops, day centres and home employment. The standard and range of services vary a great deal from authority to authority and although the welfare needs of the blind are now well catered for, in general services for other categories of severely handicapped are still inadequate.

Services for school leavers

Services for disabled school leavers merit special mention. Handicapped adolescents need extra care and attention if they are to be found suitable employment and helped to keep it. Their placing can be very difficult, particularly when their educational attainment is low, as it often is. The main source of help is the Youth Employment Service of the local authority. Careers officers visit schools to give talks on choice of employment and to interview all children nearing school leaving age. Careers officers often need to see handicapped young people several times. Their difficulties have to be discussed with teachers, parents and the school doctor, and the local Employment Medical Adviser has to be kept informed about their placement in employment to ensure a measure of continuing supervision. Some authorities now provide specialist careers officers to carry out this important task.

Appraisal of services for physically handicapped adults

The medical, social, educational and occupational needs of handicapped adults are complex and inter-related and to meet them calls for the coordination of many different services. Medical rehabilitation is provided through the hospital services, occupational rehabilitation, vocational training and resettlement services are the responsibility of the Department of Employment, while social, welfare and youth employment services are provided by local authorities. Taken together these services give a reasonably comprehensive cover, but because of failures in communication between different sectors some seriously handicapped persons (adolescents and adults) do not use to the best advantage the facilities which are available to them.

The main hindrance to the development of rehabilitation services is the low level of interest shown by hospital consultants and general practitioners in the rehabilitation and occupational needs of their patients. What is needed is a reorientation of medical thought rather than the introduction of novel techniques. In 1971 only 30 per cent of hospitals with more than 200 beds had made a named consultant responsible for rehabilitation, and there were only 131 consultants in physical medicine and rheumatology in the whole of England and Wales (89 were in the London Metropolitan area). In many hospitals physiotherapy and occupational therapy are physically separated and quite often they act as independant units. Above all, there is need for the development of assessment clinics (as described in the report of the sub-committee on Rehabilitation, 1972) to provide: focal points to bring together all services concerned in a patient's rehabilitation, both inside and outside hospital; assessment reports for the Department of Employment and the local authorities; and a safeguard against patients becoming 'lost' and failing to get the rehabilitation services they need.

FURTHER READING

Rehabilitation (1972). Report of a Sub-Committee of the Standing Medical Advisory Committee, D.H.S.S. and Welsh Office. H.M.S.O.

29 · SERVICES FOR THE MENTALLY SUBNORMAL

When the Intelligence Quotients of children in a random sample of the population are measured, the results form a continuous distribution, and they range from the low scores of grossly subnormal children at one end to the high scores of exceptionally gifted children at the other. Although a small proportion of children with low scores are identified by physical stigmata (e.g. mongols, microcephalics, cretins, etc.), the great majority have no distinguishing features. There is therefore no biological or statistical justification for drawing a line between persons of 'normal' intelligence and the mentally subnormal. The dividing line is a social one, determined by the extent to which the mental handicap interferes with the ability to lead a normal life. In particular it depends on educability and amount of care and protection required.

The Intelligence Quotient is by no means an exact or constant measure of a child's 'intelligence'. When children in a group are tested and later re-tested, the average I.Q. of the group remains much the same but the I.Q.s of individual children may vary by as much as 10 points. This is because test results are influenced by physical health, home conditions, willingness to cooperate with the examiner and many other factors. Broadly speaking, however, it can be said that most children with a score below about 70 are unlikely to derive much benefit from an ordinary school education and require special facilities. In the same way, most children with a score below about 50 are usually ineducable in the scholastic sense of the word, although many of them benefit a great deal from training designated to make the best use of their limited abilities.

Most children and adults with an I.Q. below about 50 are unable to lead independent lives. Whether the less severely handicapped among them can be looked after at home, with or without outside help, or whether they require some form of institutional care, depends on their social behaviour, home circumstances, and the supporting and training services available. These are not primarily medical matters, but, as in the case of physically handicapped children, the doctor has an important part to play in relation to ascertainment, classification and, where possible, prevention and treatment.

The Mental Health Act, 1959, brought together under a single legal code all forms of mental disorder (defined as 'mental illness, arrested or incomplete development of mind, psychopathic disorder, and any other disorder or disability of mind'). The following conditions are further defined:

(a) Severe subnormality—state of arrested or incomplete development of mind, which includes subnormality of intelligence and is of such a nature or degree that the patient is incapable of living an independent life or of guarding himself against serious exploitation or will be so incapable when of an age to do so;

(b) Subnormality—a state of arrested or incomplete development of mind (not amounting to severe subnormality) which includes subnormality of intelligence, and is of a nature or degree which requires, or is susceptible to, medical treatment or other special care or training of the patient.

In this chapter we are concerned with the needs of and services for these two groups of handicapped persons.

EVOLUTION OF SERVICES

Although for more than four hundred years it has been recognized in a general and confused way that a 'born fool' is different from a lunatic who 'hath had understanding, but by disease, grief or other accident hath lost the use of his reason', it is only during the present century that there has been any clear understanding of the distinct needs of the mentally subnormal and the mentally ill. A few asylums for 'idiots' were established by voluntary organizations during the nineteenth century, but for the most part severely subnormal children and adults who were abandoned or could not be cared for at home were placed in lunatic asylums and the only refuge for those with less severe degrees of subnormality who were unable to support themselves and could get no help from relatives or charitable sources was the general mixed workhouse.

The social inadequancy of the severely subnormal is evident and their needs are much the same in any type of society. But the difficulties and limitations of the subnormal become more obvious as the complexities of life multiply with advancing industrialization, and choice of occupation becomes increasingly dependent upon educational attainment. In England and Wales the introduction of compulsory education quickly drew attention to the fact that, apart altogether from the question of gross and unmistakable mental defect, there were many children too dull to derive much benefit from the teaching provided by ordinary schools. Gradually, special educational services developed to meet their needs, and these were codified in regulations made under the Education Act, 1944. Over the same period it became accepted that academically ineducable defectives deserve and have the right to help outside the walls of the workhouse and the mental hospital. Under the Mental Deficiency Act, 1913, local authorities were made 'mental deficiency authorities'. They became responsible for home visiting, guardianship and supervision of the subnormal in the community and for the provision of 'colonies' for the severely subnormal who for one reason or another could not be cared for at home. With the National Health Service Act, 1946, the colonies became 'mental deficiency hospitals' under the new hospital authorities, but responsibility for domiciliary care and supporting services remained with the local authorities. The Mental Health Act, 1959, greatly enlarged the local authorities' responsibilities for community care of mentally subnormal children and adults and a system of training centres and workshops was developed. With the Education(Handicapped Children) Act 1971 education authorities were required to provide education for all children regardless of mental ability, and the old Junior Training Centres are now special schools under the aegis of local education authorities who are also required to provide educational facilities in hospitals for the mentally handicapped. Responsibility for the welfare of older mentally handicapped persons now lies with the Social Services Departments of the local authorities.

CONTEMPORARY SERVICES

Educational services

Educationally subnormal children are defined as those 'who by reason of limited ability or other conditions resulting in educational retardation, require some specialized form of education wholly or partly in substitution for that normally given in ordinary schools'. They form by far the largest group of handicapped children for whom special educational services are needed (table 25). It should be noted that the definition of educational subnormality is based upon the practical consideration of educational difficulty rather than upon the theoretical concept of innate ability. Children may become educationally retarded as the result of many influences (lack of parental interest or ability, emotional disturbance, irregular school attendance, frequent change of school) as well as because of limited intellectual ability. A few children are educationally retarded in relation only to certain subjects, such as arithmetic or reading, and have an average or above average grasp of the rest of the school curriculum. The provision of educational services to meet such varied needs is clearly a complex matter and includes individual attention and special classes in ordinary schools (many backward children are in fact accommodated in the slowest stream in their schools) as well as special schools.

The special schools, about one-third of which are residential, have the great advantage of classes small enough to permit an individual as well as a group approach. The teaching is focused upon the need to help the mentally backward to acquire the minimum amount of knowledge and basic skills needed to cope with some of the complexities of modern life. The decision to send a child to a special school is not taken lightly. In an ordinary school a dull child may become duller and drift into delinquency as a result of attempting to compete with his brighter classmates, but attending a special school unfortunately still carries some stigma. For the border-line case it is only when there are serious behaviour or home difficulties (and children with an intellectual handicap tend to receive less sympathy and understanding both at school and at home than children with almost any other type of disability) that admission to a special school is considered. The decision rests upon consultation between educational psychologist, school medical officer, teacher and parents and on general assessment of social adjustment and abilities, as well as on standard intelligence and performance tests. The more seriously retarded child presents no problem and early admission to a special school is usually called for.

All but the most grossly defective children have some abilities and aptitudes which with patience and understanding can be developed, and many who at one time would have been declared untrainable are now being helped to develop fully their limited abilities in preparation for adult life in the community. These children are given training in personal cleanliness, drawing, painting and other handwork. The aim is also to teach them to grasp the essentials for ordinary living: the rudiments of road safety; the handling of money; the buying of clothing and food; and the use of public transport, post office, and health services.

Adult training centres, workshops and hostels

Young people from schools for the educationally subnormal need a continuing educational programme to adapt them to the social needs and demands of adult life and to prepare them for work in a sheltered workshop, or, possibly, for a place in open industry. Older subnormal persons require sheltered work in an environment where attention can be paid to their social needs. Local authorities are responsible for providing these facilities. The purpose is to get away from the traditional occupational therapy at one time provided in hospitals for the mentally subnormal and to provide in its place productive work and realistic preparation for life in the community. Many centres undertake contract work for the local authority (for example, a laundry service for homes, clinics and day nurseries) or for private firms in the district.

It is now clear that many patients in hospitals for the mentally subnormal do not need to be there, for they do not require medical supervision or nursing care. If parents and relatives are able with the help of local authority services to provide the social support they need, the best place for them is at home. To meet the needs of those who have no homes or whose homes are unsuitable, local authorities are beginning to provide residential accommodation. About 1,700 mentally subnormal children and adults now live in local authority hostels and homes, but the demand for such accommodation still greatly exceeds the supply.

Mental subnormality hospitals

In England and Wales there are about 160,000 mentally subnormal persons under statutory care and protection. Of these 60,000 are in mental-subnormality hospitals, the rest (100,000) are living in the community under local authority supervision or guardianship. (Supervision involves regular visits from the social services department; guardianship has a legal meaning and implies stricter supervision by an approved person who acts in loco parentis.) However well developed local authority services may become, hospital care will always be needed for some subnormal and many severely subnormal children and adults. In the past the isolation of these hospitals and their separation from the main stream of medicine and nursing could be held responsible for their low standards of care, overcrowding, lack of equipment and shortage of staff. For the first 20 years of the National Health Service little was done to improve the situation; mental subnormality hospitals remained neglected, overcrowded and underfinanced. Since about 1970, partly as the result of public disclosures of the deplorable conditions in some of the hospitals, there has been a move to remedy the worst of the deficiencies created by years of neglect. Much more capital is being invested in the services. New buildings are being erected, old buildings are being renovated to make them more suitable for patient care and improved opportunities for staff training are being provided. The move towards informal admissions, outpatient clinics, day patient facilities, industrial therapy units and hospital schools provided by local authorities is also helping to raise the standards of care.

APPRAISAL OF SERVICES

Out of date buildings and shortage of trained personnel, equipment and accommodation are complaints that can be made about many medical and social services. They can be made with particular force about services for the mentally subnormal. At the present time there are 10,000 educationally subnormal children waiting for places in special schools, more than one sixth of the number already attending. In spite of the emphasis now placed on community care, and the increasing provision by local authorities of training centres, workshops and hostels, the position is equally serious with regard to accommodation for the more severely subnormal in need of care and protection. Hospitals for the mentally subnormal, with over 60,000 patients in residence are still overcrowded and have 5,000 patients on their waiting lists, many of whom are classified as urgent.

The pressure on accommodation in special schools reflects in part the general shortage of teachers and classrooms in ordinary schools. With larger schools, smaller classes, and more teachers, it is possible that fewer border-line children would need to be referred to special schools. But pressure on accommodation in special schools comes from below as well as from above. Although the incidence of mental subnormality is not rising (it may even be falling slightly), with the decline of perinatal, infant and preschool death rates many more subnormal children are now living to school age.

As local authorities extend and strengthen their community services, it seems reasonable to expect that the need for hospital accommodation will be reduced. Nevertheless, particularly with an ageing population, there will continue to be a substantial demand for hospital care.

In conclusion we may ask if the prospect of advances in understanding of the aetiology of mental subnormality offers any hope for a reduction of its incidence by prevention or treatment. For the most part mental defect is no more than an expression of man's biological variability. But in a proportion of cases gross mental defect is due to more specific causes such as biochemical or chromosomal abnormalities. Knowledge of some of these causes (for example phenylketonuria), already permits the application of preventive or curative measures; and of a few others it is sufficient to sustain the hope that sooner or later it may be possible to do so. On present knowledge, however, it seems unlikely that medical intervention will have a significant effect on more than a small proportion of all cases of mental retardation and the problem will remain at almost its present size. Indeed, medical advances may to some extent exacerbate it. Subnormal children, especially those in institutions, are particularly vulnerable to infectious disease. With the introduction of chemotherapy, antibiotics and effective preventive inoculation, subnormal individuals who at one time would have died in infancy now survive into adult life. (This is strikingly evident in relation to mongolism.) And as the chances of survival improve, an increasing number of defectives in the community will outlive the parents and relatives who have looked after them and will need institutional care in later life.

30 · SERVICES FOR THE MENTALLY ILL

In the preceding chapter we discussed the medical and social needs of persons with mental subnormality (incomplete development of the mind manifested before adult life). We now turn to the needs of patients with mental illness (temporary or permanent disturbance of the mind, characterized by behaviour and reasoning disorders and usually occurring in adult life). Some indication of the magnitude of the problem is provided by the fact that in 1971 about 30 per cent of the hospital beds in England and Wales were set aside for such patients.

It is often difficult to draw a line between health and somatic disease. It is even more difficult to decide where mental health ends and mental illness begins. A person is thought to be mentally ill if his behaviour deviates substantially from some generally recognized but ill-defined pattern regarded as normal. But in the general population the range of behaviour extends from strict adherence to the locally accepted norms, through eccentricity and the hinterland of psychoneurosis, to the extremity of gross psychosis. Moreover, standards of acceptable social behaviour vary enormously from one civilization to another, from one community to another and even from group to group within the same community; so that behaviour which in one society would be accepted as no more than amiable eccentricity, in another may be considered to require medical treatment or even compulsory detention. Dostoevsky describes an uncle who used to shoot a gun from his window at passersby he did not like, and who sometimes opened a trapdoor to spit on a sleeping relative who also had incurred his displeasure. In Pre-Revolution Russia these practices were not apparently regarded as particularly remarkable. What determines the significance of abnormal behaviour is the extent to which it interferes with ability to lead a life acceptable as tolerably normal in the context of its social surroundings. This is also true of physical handicap; but in the case of mental illness there is the added complication that some degree of control or physical restraint may be needed, either for the patient's own sake or for the sake of others, and it may have to be imposed without the patient's full understanding or consent.

The custodial aspect of care for mentally ill people has largely determined the nature of the services which have evolved to meet their needs, and in spite of the advances of the past thirty or forty years it is still of some importance. For the sake of the patient, and sometimes of his family and the community, the more severe forms of psychiatric illness usually require hospital admission. In general, however, whether a patient can be cared for at home depends to a considerable extent on social circumstances. This is hardly less true today, when quite elaborate forms of therapy can be given in outpatient clinics or day hospitals, than it was when George III at Windsor Castle endured treatment by beating, purging and straight-jacket restraint.

EVOLUTION OF SERVICES

The history of services for the mentally ill is long and complicated. Three broad phases are discernible.

Until about the end of the eighteenth century the public attitude towards madness was one of superstitious fear, engendered by the belief that it was due to demonic possession. Lunatics were treated with deliberate brutality. The rich were incarcerated in private mad houses, the poor died in jails and workhouses.

It has been said that the devil himself helped the first reforms along by moving into Royalty. Certainly George III's death saw the beginning of a more humane approach, and during the nineteenth century many public lunatic asylums were built. Although by modern standards patients were cruelly treated, the cruelty was not malicious, but was due to ignorance. Throughout the century the main concern of reformers was to provide legal safeguards against the dangers of wrongful compulsory detention.

Since the beginning of the twentieth century advances in psychological medicine have resulted in a change in attitude towards mental illness, and the emphasis has shifted from compulsory segregation to early diagnosis, active treatment and social rehabilitation.

The nineteenth century preoccupation with the legal aspects of admission to lunatic asylums culminated in the Lunacy Act, 1890. Under this Act certification was so hemmed in with legal safeguards that a patient was likely to be admitted to an asylum only as a last resort when his illness had reached an advanced stage. So long as both the general public and the medical profession regarded lunacy as irreversible, this was of little consequence. But from the end of the nineteenth century the work of Charcot, Freud, Jung, Adler, and others suggested that at least some forms of mental illness were treatable, an impression substantially reinforced by the study of psycho-neurotic behaviour (shell shock) during the First World War. Society began to treat lunatics as sick persons not dangerous animals; but most people still regarded with fear and repugnance the legal formality of certification and the locked doors of the lunatic asylums. The Mental Treatment Act, 1930, introduced the idea of voluntary and temporary admission for treatment; it emphasized the need for psychiatric out-patient clinics, and underlined the new approach by using the expressions 'mental hospital' and 'mental illness' in place of 'lunatic asylums' and 'lunacy'. Movement in the direction of early treatment and social rehabilitation was carried several stages further by the Mental Health Act, 1959, with its emphasis on community services. It insisted that the great majority of patients suffering from mental illness shall be admitted to and treated in hospitals in the same way as patients with any other illness, and that compulsory admission and detention should be a last resort.

CONTEMPORARY SERVICES

Mentally ill patients, or their relatives, usually seek advice in the first instance from their general practitioners. If a doctor considers one of his patients to be in need of specialized treatment he seeks the opinion of a consultant psychiatrist, who sees the patient at a psychiatric clinic or, if the illness is severe, in the patient's home. If the psychiatrist thinks that hospital treatment is advisable, he can arrange for the patient to be admitted to a general or mental hospital, or to attend a psychiatric clinic or a day hospital. Occasionally the general practitioner is faced with a psychiatric emergency. In this case, he can call on the help of the Social Services Department of the local authority to arrange compulsory admission to hospital.

The Mental Health Act, 1959, greatly simplified the machinery for compulsory admission. An application is founded on the written recommendations of two medical practitioners that detention in hospital is necessary in the patient's own interests or for the protection of others. (One of the recommending practitioners must be approved as having special experience in mental disorders.) The application is made by the nearest relative of the patient or by the Social Services Department. Compulsory admission and detention may not normally exceed twentyeight days. In cases of great urgency one medical recommendation is sufficient, but the application is then valid for only seventy-two hours.

In-patient care

Between 1954 and 1971 the average number of psychiatric patients resident in hospital in England and Wales fell from 152,000 to 103,000, a decline of 32 per cent. Over the same period the number of patients admitted to mental hospitals rose from 77,000 to 178,000, an increase of 130 per cent. These trends provide a striking illustration of the way in which the pattern of care in mental hospitals is changing. On the one hand many long stay patients are being rehabilitated and returned to the community; on the other hand there is a great increase in numbers of readmissions and of patients in the early stages of mental illness.

So far as possible first admissions are accommodated in new or modernized admission wards with access to the wide range of facilities demanded by present day methods of investigation and treatment. At the same time there is a growing tendency to admit patients with less severe forms of mental illness to psychiatric wards in district general hospitals. Standards of care and treatment for the long stay patient are also rapidly improving. There are still some aggressive and difficult patients who need heavy sedation and close supervision; but in all hospitals most doors, and in some hospitals all doors, have been unlocked, and patients have much greater freedom of movement in and about the buildings, which are consequently less prison-like. It is now clear that modern drugs and an imaginative programme of recreation and occupational rehabilitation can produce so much improvement in the behaviour of long stay patients that many of them are able to return to their homes, sometimes to work.

This improvement is not achieved merely by providing work on the wards. Day rooms and dining rooms are more cheerful and more homely; facilities are provided for physical training, for watching and playing games, for dances and entertainment of various kinds; and more realistic occupational rehabilitation is being offered in workshops inside and outside the hospital buildings. Patients who improve are able to go home for the day or the weekend, and relatives are encouraged to accept them back. A period in an industrial rehabilitation unit, if there is one in the area, can sometimes hasten the slow process of return to the community.

Psychiatric clinics and day hospitals

Psychiatric clinics, providing full facilities for diagnosis and treatment by both physical and psychological methods, are now generally available, and many day hospitals have been established. Their purpose is to enable patients to maintain family ties while undergoing investigation and treatment. In this way admission to hospital can often be avoided, to the patient's benefit (in the public mind there is still some stigma attached to admission) and to the benefit of the community (clinics and day hospitals are easier to run and less expensive than residential institutions).

After-care services

In 1971 over 100,000 patients were discharged from mental hospitals in England and Wales, and another 200,000 attended psychiatric clinics and day hospitals for the first time. The problem of providing after-care services for such a large population is formidable. It is not made easier by the division of responsibility between Area Health Authorities, local authorities and the Department of Employment, or by the acute shortage of social workers. Social workers attempt to ensure that patients fit to leave hospital have a suitable home to go to before they are discharged and help patients discharged from hospital to adjust to family life and employment. Rehabilitation and vocational training services are available for them through the Department of Employment. But coordination of these varied services is difficult to achieve and the results are still far from satisfactory. In particular there is need for many more sheltered workshops and for more hostels in which patients who have no homes can live under supervision and from which they can go out to work.

THE INCIDENCE OF MENTAL ILLNESS

In view of the difficulty of defining mental illness, it is not surprising that knowledge of the amount of illness in the community is very incomplete. In England and Wales at the present time there are about 100,000 patients in mental hospitals and 200,000 new cases and three times as many old cases attending psychiatric clinics every year. This suggests that the prevalence of mental illness severe enough to warrant detention in hospital or out-patient investigation and treatment is at least 18 per 1,000 of the population. This estimate takes no account of the large number of patients with mental illness who are under the care of their general practitioners nor of the large number of old people with gross mental disturbances who are in long-stay and geriatric hospitals or are being cared for at home. In addition there is an unknown but certainly a large amount of mental ill health in the population which never comes to medical attention but causes a great deal of sickness, absence from work, and personal and family distress. Estimates of the proportion of patients seen by general practitioners who are suffering from some form of psychiatric disorder (mental subnormality, dementia, psychosis, neurosis, psychosomatic conditions, organic illnesses with a psychological overlay and personality disorder) vary between 10 and 25 per cent and it has been suggested that as much as one third of all long-term absence from work is due to psychoneurotic conditions.

It is hardly necessary to point out that if knowledge of present day incidence of mental illness is incomplete, estimates of past and future trends are even less reliable. A few general observations are permissible. The amount of mental illness attributable to acute and chronic infection, malnutrition, alcohol and toxic hazards in industry is considerably less today than it was a hundred or even fifty years ago. For example, in the mental hospitals in England and Wales during the present century the proportion of male admissions due to syphilis has declined from about one in five to less than one in 200. On the other hand mental illness associated with drug dependence is increasing. We can be less confident about the trend of those forms of mental illness whose aetiology is still obscure: schizophrenia, manic-depressive psychosis and psycho-neurosis. It is possible that there has been some reduction in the incidence of overt schizophrenia (still responsible for one-fifth of all hospital admissions) as the result of social improvements, for breakdown from this condition is commoner in poor than in favourable social circumstances. There is some evidence, however, that manic-depressive psychosis is becoming more frequent, particularly among women, and it is certain that in the ageing population the amount of mental disease associated with advanced age is rising. It is also said that the stresses of urban and industrial life have been responsible for an increase in the amount of psychoneurotic and psychosomatic illness in the community, but there is little evidence to support this view.

APPRAISAL OF SERVICES

The low standard of care in many mental hospitals is one of the most unsatisfactory features of the contemporary medical services. This deficiency has its origin in the historical circumstances which divided mental from other hospitals. Almost all of them were built more than fifty years ago, many more than a century ago, and they were designed not to treat illness, but to protect society from the embarrassing and occasionally dangerous behaviour of the insane. Lunatic asylums, built as detention barracks, serve now in part as hospitals, in part as hostels and in part as rehabilitation centres. Their wards are badly designed, inadequately equipped and far too large for modern methods of treatment. Their separation from other hospitals has isolated them and adds to the difficulty of attracting doctors and nurses.

Some hope for the future is offered by the striking decline in the number of occupied mental hospital beds, due to the discharge of many long-stay patients and the shorter average duration of stay among new admissions and re-admissions. There is some prospect that with the help of modern therapy, an expansion of still inadequate community services (day hospitals, hostels, sheltered workshops and local authority domiciliary supervisory services) and the introduction of psychiatric units into district general hospitals, there will be a further decline in the demand for mental hospital beds.

In the past treatment has been less effective in mental illness than in almost any other branch of medicine. The value of modern therapy is difficult to assess, but it is undoubtedly more effective than ever before. It is impossible to say how often psychotherapy is effective, but it is so time consuming that an insignificant proportion of the large number of psychoneurotic persons in the population can be treated by this method. The contribution of modern therapy to the control of psychosis is more concrete. In selected cases (particularly in patients with manic depressive psychosis) electro-convulsive therapy, lithium and the tricyclic antidepressants often produce an immediate and sometimes a dramatic improvement although relapse is not uncommon. There are now many drugs which have valuable sedative effects on patients in a stage of psychotic excitement, and chemical sedation has replaced the padded cell and the straight-jacket. In spite of these therapeutic advances, it seems likely that for some time to come services for the mentally ill will depend for the most part on maintainance therapy, care, protection and social rehabilitation rather than on cure.

31 · SERVICES FOR THE ELDERLY

The twentieth century has seen a great increase in the number and proportion of old people in the population. At the beginning of the twentieth century the high birth rates and high death rates of the nineteenth century produced a population with a concentration in the younger age groups. The decline in the birth rate from 1870 until just before the Second World War and the reduction of mortality from infectious disease and malnutrition in childhood and young adult life have subsequently modified population structure to produce a middle aged spread and a much greater proportion of old people (figure 7). In England and Wales in 1901 there were 1,518,000 people aged 65 or more (4·7 per cent of the population). At the 1971 census the number was 6,398,000 (13·1 per cent of the population); four million were over seventy years of age and more than a million over eighty years of age (at this age there were more than two women to every man). The expectation of life at birth in 1971 was 69·0 for males and 75·3 for females and for the first time in our history considerably more than half of all our live born infants can expect to live through to retirement. Although there have always been old people, senescence as a normal feature of life is new.

Injury, mental illness, neoplasm, arthritis and degenerative vascular states are common in the elderly, but they are not peculiar to old age. It is not because of special pathology that health and social services for old people need special consideration, although multiple pathology is certainly much commoner in old people than in young and middle aged adults. It is because the pathology of old age is associated with retirement from work, failing physical and mental powers, social isolation and a terminal illness, often preceeded by a long period of incapacity. Against this background we shall look briefly at the history of services for old people and describe in more detail the services now available to them.

EVOLUTION OF SERVICES

Public provision of personal medical and social services for old people is of very recent origin. In the nineteenth century except for a few homes provided by charitable and religious organizations, the only refuge for destitute old people and sick old people with no one to look after them was the general mixed workhouse along with the destitute of all ages. Many workers subscribed to friendly societies which provided them with small weekly payments during sickness or disablement while they were of working age and their relatives with a death grant when they died, but medical attention in old age was very rarely included among the benefits. The introduction in 1908 of a noncontributory pension of five shillings per week for needy persons over seventy years of age and in 1911 (National Health Insurance Act) of general practitioner care for old people who had paid the necessary insurance contributions during their working lives helped a small proportion of those in need. But the great majority of old people who were urgently in need of medical and nursing attention and had no children or other relatives to look after them were admitted to Poor Law Hospitals, notorious for their low standard of care. The transfer of the Poor Law Institutions to local authorities in 1929 had less effect on the low standards of hospital care than might have been expected. However, progressive authorities, following the example of charitable organizations, began to provide accommodation for well old people in residential houses and to convert the best of the hospital accommodation into general hospitals.

The less satisfactory Poor Law Institutions although transferred to local authorities remained unchanged until in 1948 (under the National Health Service Act) they became the responsibility of the newly created Regional Hospital Boards as hospitals for the chronic sick. At the same time, also under the National Health Service Act, old people, like all other members of the population, became entitled to the services of a general practitioner free of charge and, at the discretion of their general practitioner, to specialist advice and hospital care as required. Under the same act the home nursing, domestic help, health visitor and other care and after care services which local authorities were empowered to provide became available for old persons who needed them. Post war social security legislation has provided retirement pensions for all, with supplementary benefits if resources are insufficient to meet basic needs. This has removed from old people's lives the threat of financial destitution although many still have an unsatisfactorily low standard of living. Finally under the Local Authorities Social Services Act, 1970, local authorities have been made responsible for providing comprehensive social services for the care of the elderly (and other persons in need of help and support). This is implemented through their Social Services Committees and the Directors of Social Services.

CONTEMPORARY SERVICES

For a number of reasons the provision of services for the elderly presents a difficult and confusing problem. First, it is now usual to define the elderly as those aged 65 years and over and geriatrics as the branch of medicine dealing with persons of this age group. But there is nothing physiologically or medically significant about the 65th birthday. At one time old age was defined physiologically—men and women were old when they were no longer able to work. Today it is defined chronologically in terms of the age at which insured men become entitled to draw their retirement pensions. But many men and women remain physically fit and mentally alert until long past their seventieth birthdays. And on the other hand about 40 per cent of patients in the medical wards of general hospitals and in mental hospitals are over 65, while about 10 per cent of patients admitted to geriatric assessment and long-stay units are under 65. Second, whether old people who are ill or have become severely disabled are admitted to hospital or remain at home is determined more by their social circumstances and the availability of supporting services than by medical diagnosis. Third, the type of hospital to which an old person is admitted (general hospital, mental hospital, long-stay hospital, geriatric assessment unit or psychogeriatric unit) depends as much on the availability of beds in the area and on the attitudes of the general practitioners and their relationship with local consultants as on medical and nursing needs. Finally the administrative separation of health services from local authority services gives rise to difficulties in what, so far as old people are concerned, is a continuum of medical and social needs.

Area Health Authority Services

Area Health Authorities are responsible under the National Health Service Acts for providing domiciliary medical and nursing services and out-patient and in-patient hospital services for old people as for all other members of the community. However, there are certain features of these services that deserve special mention.

Domiciliary health services

Less than 5 per cent of people over 65 years of age are in geriatric units, mental hospitals and old peoples' homes. Of the 95 per cent of the elderly living in their own homes or the homes of relatives or friends, many are ill and disabled. This places a great burden on relatives and makes heavy demands on domiciliary health and social services. General practitioners provide medical attention and can obtain domiciliary or out-patient consultant advice when they think it is needed. They can call on district nurses, now often attached to group practices, for skilled and semi-skilled nursing services and on a wide range of local authority and voluntary welfare services (see below), although these still vary greatly in quality and availability from area to area. In the past, domiciliary medical services were concerned with medical crises, with acute illnesses and exacerbations of chronic illnesses as they arose. Old people are sometimes reluctant to seek medical advice through fear of hospital admission, and they are often ignorant of the welfare services that they can call on for support. General practitioners are now well aware that early mobilization of medical nursing and social services can delay the onset of dependency in old age, and health visitors, with their open access to the homes of practitioners' patients, are in a key position to detect and draw attention to old peoples' medical and social needs.

Hospital services

Many sick old people are admitted to and treated in the medical and surgical wards of general hospitals and in mental hospitals. But most teaching and district general hospitals now also have geriatric departments or geriatric assessment units. The diseases of old age are in themselves no different from the diseases of middle life, but old people much more often have multiple pathology, in their illnesses social complications are the rule rather than the exception, and they need special facilities for rehabilitation if they are to be returned to their homes. In addition a domiciliary visit by the geriatrician can sometimes avert hospital admission with the help of outpatient rehabilitation, day hospital care and supporting social services. Day hospitals, attached to and usually within the grounds of the main hospital, permit physically and sometimes mentally infirm old people to continue to live at home while receiving hospital care during the day time. Patients are brought to the day hospital by ambulance in the morning and returned home in the evening for one or more days a week. In the unit they are under medical supervision and can be given nursing attention, physiotherapy and occupational therapy. Geriatric departments also enable relief to be given to relatives when the burden of home care has become too heavy by arranging for geriatric patients to be admitted temporarily or intermittently to the wards. However, despite all these improved facilities, there are still many old people who require long-stay care. Attempts are being made to improve the quality of care in long stay hospitals. Many of the large overcrowded wards have been divided into smaller units and buildings have been modernized, so far as this is possible in nineteenth century hospitals and Poor Law buildings. But the Hospital Advisory Service, set up by the Department of Health and Social Security in 1969 and given as its first task the examination of long-stay hospitals, reported that the care of patients in them is still far from satisfactory. The separation of long-stay hospitals from the mainstream of medicine and their out of date and unsuitable buildings makes them unattractive places to work in and, therefore, difficult to staff. And although the patients in long-stay hospitals are not nearly so ill assorted as the patients in the old Poor Law Institutions, they are still very mixed in respect of their need for medical and nursing care—there are ambulant patients and permanently bedfast patients, incontinent patients and patients with senile dementia, patients with acute illness and patients with chronic and progressively disabling illness.

Local authority and voluntary services

Local authorities, through their social services committees, have statutory responsibility for providing comprehensive social services, and as part of their remit they are responsible for the care of the elderly. Many of the services they now provide were originally introduced by voluntary agencies, and voluntary organizations continue to provide services to supplement those of the local authorities and to pioneer new methods of meeting unsatisfied needs. The voluntary services are provided by many different organizations but are coordinated centrally by the National Old People's Welfare Council and locally by Old People's Welfare Committees.

Old people's homes

Residential accommodation is provided for elderly people who are in need of hospital care but are unable to live independent lives in the community because of frailty and increasing infirmity. Residents make a contribution to the cost, a general practitioner provides medical attention and a resident matron and her staff look after residents with short-term illnesses. An increasing number of these homes are new buildings, specially designed with separate or twin bedrooms, several small lounges and television, washing and ironing rooms. Other homes have been established by adapting large old houses, but these are often inconvenient and difficult to run even after extensive structural alterations have been made. Some homes are still in buildings constructed under the nineteenth century Poor Law and these are usually very unsatisfactory. The demand for places in old people's homes greatly exceeds the supply and with the shortage of suitable building sites, the rising cost of building and the shortage of trained staff it is likely to continue so.

Housing for old people

The demand for places in old people's homes and for geriatric day-hospital and in-patient care is augmented by the unsatisfactory housing in which so many old people live (houses with dangerous staircases, inadequate heating and awkwardly placed cupboards, sinks, baths and lavatories), and all local authorities now provide some special housing for elderly people. This varies in type from area to area—for example in large towns flatlets may be built with central heating, all accommodation on one floor and specially designed kitchens, lavatories and sitting baths, and in less populous areas small bungalows may be grouped near a shopping centre and other amenities. Some authorities are experimenting with groups of flats or bungalows with a restaurant and a resident warden.

Supporting services in the home

The most valuable of these is the Home Help Service. This enables many elderly people to continue to live at home who otherwise would have to be admitted to an old people's home or even to a geriatric hospital. The home help visits the home two or three times a week for about four hours at a time. She helps with the housework, does the shopping and prepares a meal. Another useful service, pioneered by the Women's Royal Voluntary Service, is 'Meals-on-Wheels'. Clinical degrees of malnutrition are quite common among very old people, especially those living alone. This is due to a combination of factors including poverty, lack of facilities for storing, preparing and cooking food and, sometimes, indifference. Hot cooked meals are delivered in insulated containers direct to the homes of such old people for a very modest charge. Other services which should be mentioned are laundry services (invaluable where an incontinent old person is being nursed at home), night sitters who undertake to sit up all night with sick old people to give exhausted relatives a night's rest (these are in very short supply) and 'good neighbour' schemes whereby someone living near an isolated and infirm old person agrees to help with the shopping, cooking and housework.

Other services

Various voluntary organizations and some local authorities help old people in other ways. For example there are luncheon clubs where hot meals are brought from a central kitchen to a suitable building in the neighbourhood, old people's clubs, day centres, handicraft centres and rest centres to combat social isolation, free transport for visiting friends and relatives, and day outings and special holiday arrangements.

APPRAISAL OF SERVICES

The purpose of most of the services we have described is to ensure that no old person enters hospital or fails to return home after completion of treatment for lack of any service which the community can reasonably be expected to provide. This is both a humane and a sensible objective—humane because, understandably, most old people want to live in their own homes, and sensible because the problem of caring for the aged sick and infirm would become unmanageable if the whole responsibility were placed on public institutions. But inadequacies in day hospital, out-patient and supporting domiciliary services are already imposing a very heavy burden on those looking after the extremely old at home. For example a recent survey has shown that a large number of bedfast incontinent old people are being cared for by middle aged and elderly relatives with no help from district nurse, laundry or other service. Sometimes this is because of ignorance about the existence of supporting services, but more often it is because the local services are inadequate. The number of people reaching extreme old age (however defined) is increasing year by year, and among the very old the prevalence of causes of dependency is high (immobility, incontinence, dementia, deafness and blindness). Local authority and voluntary services are already overburdened and even if they are greatly expanded it will still be impossible to keep many of these dependent old people at home. It is clear that to provide them with a reasonable standard of care there will need to be a considerable increase in the number of geriatric hospital beds. For example, over the age of 75 the prevalence of a degree of senile dementia requiring constant attention is about 15 per cent. This will mean at least an additional 40,000 cases in the population in ten years' time and to cater for only 10 per cent of them in hospital will require 4,000 more beds. Indeed, a substantial increase in the number of geriatric and above all psychogeriatric beds is required now if even the present level of need is to be met.

32 · INTERNATIONAL HEALTH SERVICES

Spread out across the world today is a panorama of our own health history. Less than twelve hours from London it is possible to step from a plane into an environment which presents for the local inhabitants risks of premature death from infection and malnutrition that have not existed in the British Isles since the eighteenth century. There are parts of Africa and South East Asia where the birth rate and death rates are still almost completely uncontrolled: infant mortality is over 200 and expectation of life at birth is less than 30 years. Elsewhere a rapid reduction of mortality from infectious disease is causing the explosion of population which occurred in the West in the nineteenth century. And in a country such as Sweden it is possible to see even more clearly than at home the health problems that remain when the threat of infection, largely associated with the existence of poverty, has almost been eliminated.

Modern methods of communication constantly bring these matters to public attention. Moreover, speed of transport has so reduced the time of travel between countries that the risk of spread of epidemic disease has been greatly increased. Within the incubation period of smallpox a plane can travel many times around the world and in a few hours it can transport the vector of yellow fever, the mosquito Aedes aegypti, from Africa to India. Self interest as well as humanity makes national health a matter of international concern.

Until recently the only international health problem of general interest was control of the spread of epidemic disease between countries and continents. This remains an important function of international health services, but it is one that is relatively easy to perform. More difficult, and of much greater moment today, is the control of infectious disease within countries. The difficulty here lies not in lack of knowledge, but in shortage of the funds and technical resources needed if what is already known is to be applied. So far as knowledge goes, the control of most water-borne, insect-borne and food-borne disease is within reach of every country. Geography and climate sometimes favour the spread of infection by providing suitable ecological conditions for animal and insect vectors. Nevertheless during the war troops from countries with a high standard of living remained healthy in swamp, jungle and desert. Water can be purified chemically; refuse and sewage can be disposed of hygienically; the life cycle of most disease vectors can be cut short; and the number of infectious diseases for which immunization and effective therapy are available is steadily increasing.

EVOLUTION OF INTERNATIONAL HEALTH SERVICES

Although the nature of infectious disease was not elucidated until the second half of the nineteenth century, the idea of contagion has a long history, and a 'cordon sanitaire' and compulsory isolation of epidemic areas were used as far back as the seventh century. It was the devastating pandemic of bubonic plague in the fourteenth century which led to introduction of quarantine for ships and goods arriving from areas ravaged by the disease. The idea originated in the Adriatic, probably in the republic of Venice, although Ragusa (now Dubrovnik) has some claim to priority in this practice. The agreed period of isolation was forty days (quaranta), a number chosen mainly on astrological and religious grounds.

The modern international health movement also had its origins in a pandemic. The first International Sanitary Conference was convened in Paris in 1851 in an attempt to stem the tide of cholera which had ebbed and flowed across Europe for twenty years, disrupting trade and killing hundreds of thousands. An international convention for the control of that disease (and of plague and yellow fever) was drawn up, but unanimous ratification was not achieved until forty years and seven international conferences later. A common danger brought the nations together, but national interests and the limitation of scientific knowledge delayed agreement.

But the concept of a permanent international health agency had taken root, and in 1909 L'Office International d'Hygiène Publique was established in Paris 'to collect and bring to the knowledge of participating states the facts and documents of a general character which relate to public health and especially as regards infectious diseases, notably cholera, plague and yellow fever, as well as measures to combat these diseases'.

After the First World War the threat of epidemic disease (this time typhus and influenza) once again brought the nations together, and the Health Organization of the newly created League of Nations was established. During the inter-war years the interests and concern of the Health Organization ranged far beyond the control of spread of epidemic disease by quarantine and provision of an epidemiological intelligence service. Technical commissions produced valuable reports on nutrition, housing, cancer, medical and public health training, biological standardization and the standardization of pharmacopoeias and diagnostic terminology.

The Second World War called a halt to many of the activities of the Health Organization of the League of Nations, but immediately after the war there was a resurgence of interest in international health matters. In New York in 1946 the representatives of fiftyone nations adopted the draft of the constitution of the World Health Organization, creating for the first time a single international body responsible for every aspect of health. Agreement was not reached without difficulty. Of the nations represented only China and the United Kingdom signed the Constitution without reservation, and it was not until 1948 that majority approval was given and the first World Health Assembly met in Geneva.

CONTEMPORARY INTERNATIONAL HEALTH SERVICES

The World Health Organization has accepted much greater responsibility and has a far wider sphere of influence than any of the earlier bodies concerned with international health. Its stated objective is 'the attainment by all peoples of the highest possible level of health' and this is to be regarded as 'one of the fundamental rights of every human being, without distinction of race, religion, political belief, economic or social conditions'. In the Charter of W.H.O. the belief is expressed unequivocally that all 'Governments have a responsibility for the health of their peoples which can be fulfilled only by the provision of adequate health and social measures' and that 'the health of all peoples is fundamental to the attainment of peace and security ... unequal development in different countries in the promotion of health and the control of disease, especially communicable disease, is a common danger'. These are high ideals. The machinery devised for attaining them depends for the most part, not on supra national action, but on work done for, with and through governments. The services can be described conveniently under five headings.

Quarantine and epidemiological intelligence services

In the traditional field of international health work, W.H.O. has brought together and simplified the complex muddle of sanitary conventions regulating international quarantine practices in a single code, the 'International Sanitary Regulations' replaced in 1970 by the International Health Regulations. These regulations provide for international control of the spread of epidemic disease with as little interference with trade and travel as possible. They are now accepted by 145 states and territories in full and by another 22 with some reservations. A world wide epidemiological intelligence service provides immediate information about the occurrence anywhere of the major infectious diseases (plague, cholera, yellow fever, smallpox, typhus, and relapsing fever) and of other diseases such as malaria, typhoid fever poliomyelitis and influenza. Daily bulletins are put out by short wave from Geneva and weekly bulletins from a network of stations throughout the world. It should be mentioned that the expanding packet holiday market to tropical countries has greatly increased the risk of spread of some of these diseases.

Standardization services

The pace at which medical knowledge is advancing makes the need for standardization of medical terminology and of the many new and potent therapeutic agents a matter of great urgency. W.H.O. has made a notable contribution in both fields. An internationally agreed pharmacopoeia has been published, and more than a hundred laboratories in different parts of the world cooperate to establish agreed standards for biological products ranging from diphtheria antitoxin to the newer antibiotics.

The terminology and classification of disease is peculiarly difficult. Apart from language problems, which are considerable, knowledge of aetiology is incomplete; hence any classification which is to avoid a large group of conditions categorized as 'Other and Unknown' must inevitably be based in part on aetiological, in part on pathological and in part on anatomical and physiological criteria. W.H.O. has done much to clarify the position with its International Classification of Diseases, Injuries and Causes of Death of which the eighth revision

Table 28. International Statistical Classification of Diseases, Injuries and Causes of Death (8th Revision, W.H.O., 1968)

I	Infective and parasitic diseases
II	Neoplasms
III	Endocrine, nutritional and metabolic diseases
IV	Diseases of the blood and blood-forming organs
V	Mental disorders
VI	Diseases of the nervous system and sense organs
VII	Diseases of the circulatory system
VIII	Diseases of the respiratory system
IX	Diseases of the digestive system
X	Diseases of the genito-urinary system
XI	Complications of pregnancy, childbirth and the puerperium
XII	Diseases of the skin and subcutaneous tissue
XIII	Diseases of the musculoskeletal system and connective tissue
XIV	Congenital anomalies
XV	Certain causes of perinatal morbidity and mortality
XVI	Symptoms and ill-defined conditions
XVII	Accidents, poisonings and violence

was adopted in 1968. Table 28 gives the seventeen main headings under which disease, injuries and causes of death are classified in the 'I.C.D.'. The first category (Infective and Parasitic Diseases) has a firm aetiological basis. The second category (Neoplasms) is based on Pathology. The third (Endocrine System, Nutritional and Metabolic Diseases) has a physiological background. Most of the other categories are based mainly on anatomical systems, while the last (Accidents, Poisoning and Violence) brings together causes of death with legal implications. Even the first category, although tidy from an aetiological point of view, is far from comprehensive. For example, influenza and pneumonia are included under 'Diseases of the Respiratory System' and rheumatic fever under 'Diseases of the Circulatory System'.

Education, training and the dissemination of technical information

Since 1948 many thousands of fellowships have been awarded to doctors and other health workers to enable them to study and work abroad in such diverse fields as the organization of public health and preventive services, control of communicable disease, medical education, clinical medicine and the basic medical sciences. Expert committees have reported on almost every aspect of modern medicine, including the aetiology and treatment of all major infectious and non-infectious diseases, drug addiction, insecticides, mental health, medical education, the medical problems of atomic energy and the medical use of radio-isotopes.

Research activities

Over the past two decades W.H.O. has become increasingly active in initiating and supporting research. The Organization is well placed to conduct or collaborate in epidemiological and nutritional studies in differing economic, social and ecological settings. Groups of experts are convened to review specific subjects, identify gaps in knowledge and recommend appropriate research approaches to the problems uncovered. There is a network of more than 350 W.H.O. designated references centres and about the same number of national centres with whom W.H.O. collaborates. An autonomous International Agency for Research in Cancer was established by W.H.O. in 1965, sited in Lyons (France) and many scientists are employed by the Organization to work in the Institute of Nutrition of Central America and Panama, the Pan American Zoonoses Centre near Buenos Aires, the East Africa Virus Research Institute in Entebbe, Uganda, and other research institutions financed from resources external to the regular budget of W.H.O. In these and other ways the Organization has made major contributions in the evaluation of new vaccines and sera for poliomyelitis, measles, smallpox, rabies, typhoid, cholera, tuberculosis, brucellosis, leptospirosis and cysticercosis, the classification of the epidemiology of cardiovascular diseases and certain cancers as well as of many of the communicable diseases, the relationship of protein-calorie deficiencies to infective agents and the development of many biological standards and working preparations to provide baseline references for all countries.

Services to governments

W.H.O. has perhaps made its greatest contribution by providing practical aid and expert guidance to many governments to reinforce their attack upon epidemic and endemic disease and to help them to establish sanitary, health and welfare services to meet local needs and conditions. Malaria has been controlled in a number of countries and eradication programmes for its control are under way in many more. More than 25,000,000 people living in countries where yaws is endemic have been given penicillin. Endemic typhus has been blown from Afghanistan in a cloud of D.D.T. dust. And 100,000,000 young persons throughout the world have been vaccinated with B.C.G. The organization is also active in the promotion of maternal and child care services, environmental services (water supply, sewage and refuse disposal, housing standards, air pollution, etc.) and is encouraging the development of processed protein rich foods from local sources in countries where protein deficiency in infancy is a major problem.

Largely because of mass campaigns supported by W.H.O., the great world scourges of malaria, tuberculosis, yaws and the rickettsial diseases have been in retreat since the Second World War. This is a remarkable achievement. The major problems that remain are to consolidate and extend the control of disease, and to feed the large numbers of people saved from premature death. The emphasis in international health work is shifting from successful short term attacks against major epidemic and endemic diseases to the more difficult long term problem of helping governments to establish sound public health and medical services. Perhaps the most formidable obstacle is the world wide shortage of trained medical and health personnel of all categories. W.H.O. is helping to strengthen national training institutions, but the help it can give is greatly restricted by its limited financial resources. The budget at its disposal is not much more than the amount spent on municipal health programmes by many large cities in the western world.

INDEX